医药高等职业教育公共基础课程规划教材

医药英语

English for Medicine

（供医药类各专业使用）

主　编　黄光惠　周丽丽

主　审　宫　建

副主编　胡晓莉　张媛媛　钱科颖　葛　露

编　者　（以姓氏笔画为序）

宋　枫（福建卫生职业技术学院）

张媛媛（长沙卫生职业学院）

周　欢（重庆医药高等专科学校）

周丽丽（皖西卫生职业学院）

胡晓莉（山东医学高等专科学校）

钱科颖（长春医学高等专科学校）

黄光惠（福建卫生职业技术学院）

葛　露（辽宁医药职业学院）

蒋露露（湖南食品药品职业学院）

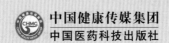
中国健康传媒集团

中国医药科技出版社

内 容 提 要

　　本教材为"医药高等职业教育公共基础课程规划教材"之一,系根据本套教材的编写指导思想和原则要求,结合专业培养目标和本课程的教学目标、内容与任务要求编写而成。本教材选取与医药相关的具有实用价值的英文素材,内容包括医学、药学和药剂师、药品分类、中药、药物研发、新药申请、药物安全性、药品营销、药品监管、医药发展趋势等,为学生学习专业课程和进一步提高医药英语奠定基础。本教材为书网融合教材,即纸质教材有机融合电子教材、教学配套资源、题库系统、数字化教学服务。

　　本教材主要供全国高职高专院校医药类各专业教学使用。

图书在版编目（CIP）数据

医药英语 / 黄光惠,周丽丽主编. —北京:中国医药科技出版社,2020.12

医药高等职业教育公共基础课程规划教材

ISBN 978 - 7 - 5214 - 2140 - 8

Ⅰ.①医…　Ⅱ.①黄…　②周…　Ⅲ.①医学－英语－高等职业教育－教材　Ⅳ.①R

中国版本图书馆 CIP 数据核字（2020）第 230663 号

美术编辑　陈君杞
版式设计　友全图文

出版　**中国健康传媒集团** | 中国医药科技出版社
地址　北京市海淀区文慧园北路甲 22 号
邮编　100082
电话　发行:010 - 62227427　邮购:010 - 62236938
网址　www.cmstp.com
规格　889×1194 mm $^1/_{16}$
印张　17
字数　482 千字
版次　2020 年 12 月第 1 版
印次　2020 年 12 月第 1 次印刷
印刷　北京市密东印刷有限公司
经销　全国各地新华书店
书号　ISBN 978 - 7 - 5214 - 2140 - 8
定价　75.00 元

获取新书信息、投稿、为图书纠错,请扫码联系我们。

出版说明

为深入贯彻《现代职业教育体系建设规划（2014—2020 年）》以及《医药卫生中长期人才发展规划（2011—2020 年）》文件的精神，满足高职高专医药院校公共基础课程培养目标的要求，不断提升人才培养水平和教育教学质量，在教育部、国家卫生健康委员会及国家药品监督管理局的领导和指导下，在本套教材建设指导委员会专家的指导和顶层设计下，中国医药科技出版社有限公司组织全国 30 余所高职高专院校及附属医疗机构近 120 名专家、教师精心编撰了医药高等职业教育公共基础课程规划教材，该套教材即将付梓出版。

本套教材共包括 12 门，主要供全国高等职业教育医药类院校各专业教学使用。

本套教材定位清晰、特色鲜明，主要体现在以下方面。

一、遵循教材编写的基本规律

本套教材编写遵循"三基、五性、三特定"的基本规律。基本理论和基本知识以"必需、够用"为度，兼顾学生终身学习能力的培养。公共基础课程是专业基础课程的基础，应该注意衔接专业基础课程教学的需要。但也注意把握好教材内容的深度和广度，不能要求大而全，以适应全国高等职业教育的需要为度，适当反映学科的新进展。

在保证教材思想性和科学性的基础上，特别强调教材的适用性与先进性。考虑到高等职业教育模式发展中的多样性，在教材的编写过程中，保障学生具备专业教学标准要求的知识和技能，适当兼顾不同院校学生的要求，以保证教材的适用性。教材的基本理论知识（如概念、名词术语等）应避免陈旧过时，要注意吐故纳新，做到科学先进，不陈旧，跟上学科发展步伐，保证内容的科学性和先进性。同时，教材应融传授知识、培养能力、提高素质为一体，重视培养学生的创新、获取信息及终身学习的能力，突出教材的启发性。

二、满足人才培养需要

教材编写应以专业培养目标为导向，满足 3 个需要（岗位需要、学教需要、社会需要）。这是编写本套教材的重要原则。

1. 岗位需要 是指教材编写应满足工作岗位所需的知识、技能、素质、心理等要求，有利于学生形成科学的思维和学习方法。

2. 学教需要 是指教材编写有利于学生学和教师教，符合学生的认知特点和教学规律。

3. 社会需要 是指教材编写应能够满足社会对学生知识和技能的要求、人文素质要求，使学生不仅能满足当前社会的要求，还具备一定的可持续发展潜力。

三、体现职教特色

高职高专教材不应该是本科教材的缩略版，应该体现职业教育的特色。

1. 以就业为导向，突出实用 高等职业教育培养的是技术技能型人才，不强调人才具有多么高的理论修养和渊博的知识，一切以生产岗位对人才能力的需求为中心，基础课程要突出素质要求，重点培养学生在岗位中必备的身体、心理、人文的素质。

2. 加强人文素养，全面提高学科素质 公共基础课程教材在强调实用的同时，也不能否定课程本身的属性和功能。公共基础课程不单是学习其他课程的基础，也是引导学生自身向高层次发展的基础，更是走向社会生活的基础。教材不仅要培养学生掌握相关的知识，还要引导学生的思想认识、道德修养、文化品位和审美情趣，注重创造力的培养，提高学生的整体素质。

3. 培养自学能力，提高职业能力 终身教育、继续教育已逐渐成为国际公认的教育理念。不会自学，就不会有自我发展和创造能力。教材是教本，教材的编写应注重把学生的自学能力培养起来，教材编写注重让学生触类旁通，举一反三，掌握学习方法，养成自学习惯。

四、多媒融合配套增值服务

纸质教材与数字教材融合，提供给师生多种形式的教学共享资源，以满足教学的需要。本套教材在纸质教材建设过程中增加书网融合内容，此外，还搭建与纸质教材配套的"在线学习平台"，增加网络增值服务内容（如课程 PPT、试题、视频、动画等），使教材内容更加生动化、形象化。

编写出版本套高质量教材，得到了全国知名专家的精心指导和各有关院校领导与编者的大力支持，在此一并表示衷心感谢。出版发行本套教材，希望受到广大师生欢迎，并在教学中积极使用本套教材，提出宝贵意见，以便修订完善，共同打造精品教材。

医药高等职业教育公共基础课程规划教材

建设指导委员会

医药高等职业教育公共基础课程规划教材

评审委员会

数字化教材编委会

主　编　黄光惠　周丽丽

副主编　胡晓莉　张媛媛　钱科颖　葛　露

编　者　（以姓氏笔画为序）

宋　枫（福建卫生职业技术学院）

张媛媛（长沙卫生职业学院）

周　欢（重庆医药高等专科学校）

周丽丽（皖西卫生职业学院）

胡晓莉（山东医学高等专科学校）

钱科颖（长春医学高等专科学校）

黄光惠（福建卫生职业技术学院）

葛　露（辽宁医药职业学院）

蒋露露（湖南食品药品职业学院）

　　《医药英语》为"医药高等职业教育公共基础课程规划教材"之一，根据公共基础课程专业培养目标和主要就业方向及医药职业能力要求，按照本套教材编写指导思想和原则要求，结合《高等职业教育英语课程教学基本要求（试用）》，由全国 8 所院校从事教学和生产一线的教师、学者悉心编写而成，皆在培养学生在职场环境下运用英语的技能，从而增强学生的就业竞争力，并为学生未来职业生涯和职业能力的可持续发展奠定坚实的基础，满足医药行业对国际化人才的需求。适用于全国高职高专院校医药类各专业教学。

　　本教材涉及医药相关的各个领域知识，内容主要包括医学、药学和药剂师、药品分类、中药、药物研发、新药申请、药物安全性、药品营销、药品监管、医药发展趋势 10 个主题。在选材上融入《国家执业药师职业资格考试大纲》（第八版，2020 年）的部分内容，并与"高等学校英语应用能力考试 PRETCO – A/B 级"和"全国高职院校技能大赛（英语口语）"对接，选取与医药相关理论知识以及在不同医药职场环境下具有实用价值的英文素材。本教材的任务是使学生在公共英语学习的基础上，掌握医药英语基本知识与技能，培养医药职场环境下英语听、说、读、写、译的能力，从而能借助词典阅读和翻译医药相关的英语业务资料，在涉外交际的业务活动中进行基本的口头和书面交流，为学习专业课程和进一步提高医药英语的应用能力奠定良好的基础。

　　本教材为"教学做一体化"教材。全书共 10 个单元，每单元教学时间设计为 6 学时，可以根据不同专业需求选择适合的内容。各单元具体内容如下：

　　单元介绍（Introduction）：总体介绍单元主题，帮助师生从整体上把握本单元的核心信息。

　　单元导入（Warming-up）：图文配对，介绍与单元主题相关、最具代表性的知识点。

　　课文 A（Reading A）：课文主要选自与医药主题相关的国内外英文刊物。其中生词和短语（Words and Expressions）以在课文中出现的顺序排列，提供简洁准确的中文释义；注释（Notes）对文中涉及的专有名词提供知识背景，对一些特别语言现象给予必要的解释。课后习题（After-reading Exercises）包括回答问题、词汇和汉译英练习。

　　听说部分（Listening & Speaking）：听力素材为单元主题相关的医药职场情境对话，题型设置参照"高等学校英语应用能力考试 PRETCO – A/B 级"。口语涉及与听力相关主题，题型设置结合"全国高职院校技能大赛（英语口语）"。

　　课文 B（Reading B）：从不同角度提供单元相关信息。其中生词和短语（Words and Expressions）以在课文中出现顺序排列。课后习题（After-reading Exercises）包括阅读理解和英译汉练习。

应用写作（Practical Writing）：参考"高等学校英语应用能力考试 PRETCO – A/B 级"的题型及部分内容，结合医药职场相关应用写作类型进行写作训练，主要通过范例学习要求学生能够仿写招聘广告、表格、求职简历、公司简介、海报、电子邮件、药品说明书、报告、商务信函、摘要等。

语法知识（Grammar Tips）：简要归纳说明英语语法，并进行复习巩固性练习。

补充阅读（Supplementary Reading）：单元主题相关的补充性阅读，可作为阅读理解练习。

词汇学习技巧（Vocabulary Tips）：分析医学术语构词特点，帮助学生提高词汇学习效率。

谚语俗语（Proverbs and Sayings）：医药相关谚语俗语，有助于了解医药相关文化。

本教材为书网融合教材，即纸质教材有机融合电子教材、教学配套资源、题库系统、数字化教学服务。

本书由福建卫生职业技术学院黄光惠和皖西卫生职业学院周丽丽担任主编。编写人员分工如下：福建卫生职业技术学院黄光惠编写第一单元及全书词汇学习技巧部分；福建卫生职业技术学院黄光惠和皖西卫生职业学院周丽丽共同编写第二单元；皖西卫生职业学院周丽丽编写第三单元；辽宁医药职业学院葛露编写第四单元；长沙卫生职业学院张媛媛编写第五单元；长春医学高等专科学校钱科颖编写第六单元；山东医学高等专科学校胡晓莉编写第七单元；湖南食品药品职业学院蒋露露编写第八单元；福建卫生职业技术学院宋枫编写第九单元；重庆医药高等专科学校周欢编写第十单元。两位主编共同拟定本书的编写提纲和编写体例，主编和副主编承担主要审稿工作。沈阳药科大学的宫建教授对全书进行全面的审阅。全体编写团队教师牺牲大量个人时间，为本书的编写付出辛勤的劳动和心血，在此表示衷心的感谢。

本书在编写过程中得到了编写团队学校领导和多位企业技术专家的支持和帮助，在此一并表示衷心的感谢！同时感谢外籍教师 Steven Hellwig 与 Katrina James 对本书英文进行审阅！

由于受编者知识所限，疏漏之处在所难免。恳请广大读者及各方面专家、学者提出宝贵意见，编者将不胜感激。

编　者

2020 年 10 月

目录

教学大纲

Unit 1

Medicine

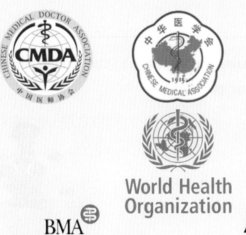

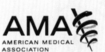

PPT

Unit Objectives

After studying this unit, you are expected to:

· master the vocabulary and technical terms related to Traditional Chinese Medicine and Western Medicine;

· understand Traditional Chinese Medicine and Western Medicine;

· know English parts of speech correctly.

And you should learn how to:

· communicate with others about diseases and Western and Eastern Medicine;

· write a job posting.

Introduction

Medicine is the science and practice of establishing the diagnosis, prognosis, treatment, and prevention of disease. Medicine encompasses a variety of health care practices evolved to maintain and restore health by the prevention and treatment of illness.

In the western world, conventional modern medicine is sometimes called Western Medicine or

Introduction

医药大学堂
WWW.YIYADDXT.COM

allopathic medicine. It involves the use of drugs or surgery, often supported by counseling and lifestyle measures. Alternative and complementary types of medicine include Traditional Chinese Medicine, acupuncture, homeopathy, herbal medicine, art therapy, and many more.

Traditional Chinese Medicine or TCM is one of the world's oldest forms of medicine. But in a world predominantly using western medical science, the popularity of Traditional Chinese Medicine is regaining popularity. Many of the principles and ancient wisdom of TCM are being integrated into holistic strategies for health today.

Warming-up

Task　Work in groups. Match the pictures to the proper statements. Then check your answers with your partner.

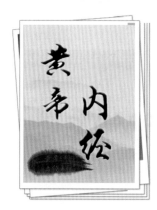

A

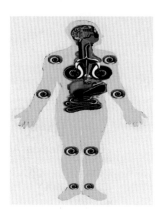

B

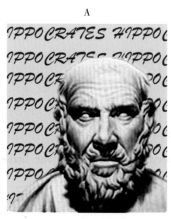

C

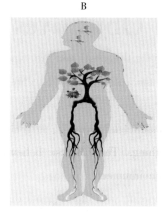

D

(　) 1. The goal of eastern medicine is to support the natural processes of the body. Health is defined as the bio-equilibrium between the body and nature.

(　) 2. The goal of western medicine is to fight symptoms and maximize performance. Health is defined as the absence of disease and body as machine with separate parts.

(　) 3. *The Yellow Emperor's Inner Classic* (*Huang Di Nei Jing*) is an ancient Chinese medical text that has been treated as the fundamental doctrinal source for Chinese medicine for more than two millennia.

(　) 4. Hippocrates, "Father of Medicine", was a Greek physician who is considered one of the most outstanding figures in the history of medicine.

Reading A

Traditional Chinese Medicine

Traditional Chinese Medicine——also often referred to as "Eastern Medicine"——originated in ancient mainland China. It dates back more than 2,500 years and has evolved and been perfected ever since. But what exactly is Traditional Chinese Medicine? An understanding of the premises of TCM starts with the underlying philosophies.

Yin and Yang

Nature is the primary hallmark of TCM. The basic premise of TCM is that our bodies are a microcosm of our surrounding world and universe. Yin and yang is the basis of Eastern science and TCM. It is the concept that opposing forces are actually complementary, essential, and need to exist in balance and harmony for optimal health. Some examples are:

· light and dark

· positive and negative

· fire and water

· good and evil

· male and female

· expanding and contracting

Think about it this way. Shadows cannot exist without light. And the premise of many modern superhero movies——good cannot exist without evil. The basic underlying premise of yin and yang in TCM is these seemingly opposite forces need to exist in balance and harmony. Harmony between yin and yang is thought to promote health. But imbalance is thought to result in disease.

Qi

Qi (pronounced "Chee"), is generally defined as the vital energy that flows through the bodies of every living thing. The Chinese believed that Qi permeated everything and linked our bodies' to the surrounding environment.

The concept of Qi is deeply rooted in Traditional Chinese Medicine. The concept was first noted in the oldest TCM scriptures, named the '*Internal Scripture*'. The concept is that vital energy circulates through our bodies in pathways referred to as meridians. Symptoms or overt illnesses are believed to be the result of blocked, disrupted, or unbalanced Qi moving through our meridians. A properly flowing Qi is believed to be responsible for many aspects of health. Thus, a major focus of TCM practices is often targeted at unblocking and allowing our Qi to properly circulate throughout our bodies.

Five Elements

"The Five Elements" or "Five Phases" consist of metal, wood, water, fire and earth. Each represents different properties, functions or appearances under which all things in the universe can be classified. This concept is used to describe interactions and relationships between all natural phenomena, including the stages of human life, and explain the functioning of the body and how it changes during health or disease.

Practitioners use a variety of protocols to treat what is believed to be at the root of an underlying health condition. These can include interventions around nutrition, diet, herbal remedies, and various mind or body practices. These treatments can include acupuncture, cupping, therapeutic massage, scraping, reflexology, bone setting, chiropractic techniques, breathing, exercise, and self-defense trainings.

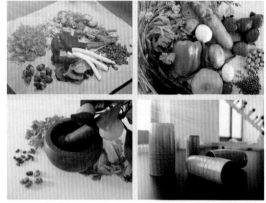

Ancient TCM concepts emphasize a natural, preventive approach. At the core of the Traditional Chinese Medicine philosophy is that corrective, preventative action can help if the right steps are taken. Traditional Chinese Medicine principles can help you strengthen your holistic health and wellness. It can guide you as you develop a healthier lifestyle that connects the pillars of physical, emotional, environmental, nutritional, and spiritual health.

(554 words)

Words and Expressions			
originate	/əˈrɪdʒɪneɪt/	vi.	发源
evolve	/iˈvɒlv/	vi.	发展；进化
premise	/ˈpremɪs/	n.	前提，假定
underlying	/ˌʌndəˈlaɪɪŋ/	adj.	潜在的；根本的
philosophy	/fəˈlɒsəfi/	n.	哲学；哲理；人生观
hallmark	/ˈhɔːlmɑːk/	n.	特点；品质证明
microcosm	/ˈmaɪkrəʊkɒzəm/	n.	微观世界；缩图
complementary	/ˌkɒmplɪˈmentri/	adj.	补足的；互补的
harmony	/ˈhɑːməni/	n.	和谐；协调
optimal	/ˈɒptɪməl/	adj.	最佳的；最理想的
positive	/ˈpɒzətɪv/	adj.	正的；阳性的
negative	/ˈnegətɪv/	n.	负的；阴性的
contract	/ˈkɒntrækt/	v.	收缩
permeate	/ˈpɜːmieɪt/	vt.	渗透，透过；弥漫
scripture	/ˈskrɪptʃə(r)/	n.	经文；（大写）圣经
meridian	/məˈrɪdiən/	n.	中医经脉；经线
symptom	/ˈsɪmptəm/	n.	[临床] 症状；征兆
overt	/əʊˈvɜːt/	adj.	明显的
disrupt	/dɪsˈrʌpt/	vt.	破坏
property	/ˈprɒpəti/	n.	性质，性能
phenomenon	/fəˈnɒmɪnən/	n.	现象（复数 phenomena）
protocol	/ˈprəʊtəkɒl/	n.	协议；方案
intervention	/ˌɪntəˈvenʃn/	n.	介入；调停

续表

herbal	/ˈɜːrdl, ˈhɜːrdl/	adj.	草药的；草本的
remedy	/ˈremədi/	n.	疗法
acupuncture	/ˈækjupʌŋktʃə(r)/	n.	针灸
cupping	/ˈkʌpiŋ/	n.	拔火罐
therapeutic	/ˌθerəˈpjuːtik/	adj.	治疗的
massage	/məˈsɑːʒ/	n.	按摩，推拿
scraping	/ˈskreipiŋ/	n.	刮痧
reflexology	/ˌriːfleksˈɒlədʒi/	n.	［心理］反射学；（按摩脚部的）反射疗法
chiropractic	/kaiərəʊˈpræktik/	n.	脊椎按摩疗法
holistic	/həʊˈlistik/	adj.	整体的
Proper Names			
TCM（Traditional Chinese Medicine）			中国传统医学，简称中医

📖 Notes

1. The basic premise of TCM is that our bodies are a microcosm of our surrounding world and universe.

中医的基本前提是，我们的身体是我们周围世界和宇宙的一个缩影。

本句含 that 引导的表语从句，通常"that"不省略，但在非正式语体中有时也可以省略。

e. g. The basic underlying premise of yin and yang in TCM is these seemingly opposite forces need to exist in balance and harmony.

中医阴阳学说的基本前提是这些看似对立的力量需要平衡和和谐地存在。

2. It is the concept that opposing forces are actually complementary, essential, and need to exist in balance and harmony for optimal health.

阴阳概念是指对立的力量实际上是互补，（互为）根本，需要在平衡、和谐中存在，以达到最佳的健康状态。

本句含 that 引导的同位语从句。对前面的名词"concept"（通常是抽象名词）起解释说明作用。常见的抽象名词有：idea, opinion, fact, evidence, question, doubt, reason, theory, belief, possibility, chance, hope, contention, finding, notion 等。

e. g. You just have no idea what you want to buy. 你自己要买什么根本没有想法。

3. The concept was first noted in the oldest TCM scriptures, named the 'Internal Scripture'.

最古老的中医典籍《内经》中最早记载这一概念。

'Internal Scripture'：《内经》是《黄帝内经》的简称。《黄帝内经》有多个英文译名，如：*The Yellow Emperor's Inner Classic*（*Huang Di Nei Jing*），*The Yellow Emperor's Canon of Medicine*，*The Yellow Emperor's Canon of Internal Medicine* 等。

4. Symptoms or overt illnesses are believed to be the result of blocked, disrupted, or unbalanced Qi moving through our meridians.

经络气滞、中断或不平衡就会产生疾病症状或明显的疾病。

"moving through our meridians" 为现在分词短语作后置定语修饰 Qi，相当于定语从句"which moves through our meridians"。

5. "Five Elements" or "Five Phases"：五行。

对于"五行"的译法争议较大。译词 elements 可解释为"要素",中医中的五行是五种物质,其变化运动构成了人体阴阳变化。但 elements 是静态的,并不很准确。phases 的意思是"形态",主要是指物理、化学上的物质形态,与中医理论中的五行概念也有一定的差别。按照中国古典哲学的理念,"五行"的"行"应该是一个动词,即 movement 或 interaction。但将"五行"译为 five elements 是一个最为普遍的译法。

6. Each represents different properties, functions or appearances under which all things in the universe can be classified.

五种物质代表不同的功能、属性或性状,宇宙间万物并以此进行归类。

"under which…"为"介词 + 关系代词"结构引导的定语从句,此处关系代词只能用 which (指物) 或 whom (指人)。

e. g. The little girl is reading a book, in which there are many cartoons.

小女孩正在读一本有许多卡通图画的书。

After-reading Exercises

Task 1　Answer the following questions according to the text.

1. What are the basic philosophies of Traditional Chinese Medicine?

_____

2. How does the concept of Yin and Yang explain the causes of health and disease?

_____

3. Which classic of TCM first noted the concept of Qi?

_____

4. How can all things in the universe be classified according to the Five Elements?

_____

5. Can you tell the benefits of TCM according to the text?

_____

Task 2　Match the words (1-10) to the Chinese meanings (a-j).

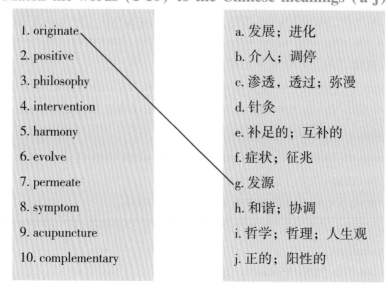

1. originate	a. 发展;进化
2. positive	b. 介入;调停
3. philosophy	c. 渗透、透过;弥漫
4. intervention	d. 针灸
5. harmony	e. 补足的;互补的
6. evolve	f. 症状;征兆
7. permeate	g. 发源
8. symptom	h. 和谐;协调
9. acupuncture	i. 哲学;哲理;人生观
10. complementary	j. 正的;阳性的

Task 3   Fill in each blank with the proper form of the word or phrase given in brackets.

1. Your cover letter should _____, not duplicate your resume. (complementary)

2. The pain _____ from a point in his right thigh. (originate)

3. "Our hope is that if we feed blueberry juice to a child with this type of tumour, we can _____ and shrink the tumour before it becomes a big problem," said Gordillo. (intervention)

4. So it is possible that these _____ will not finally go until your nervous system is in a better state. (symptom)

5. He was thrown out of the Olympic team after testing _____ for drugs. (positive)

Task 4   Translate the following sentences into English using the words or phrases you have learned in this unit.

1. 中医可追溯到 2500 多年前，从那时起不断发展完善。(evolve)

_____

2. 中国人认为，气渗透于万物，并使我们的身体与周围环境联系在一起。(permeate)

_____

3. 阴阳和谐就可以促进健康。(promote)

_____

4. 五行由金、木、水、火、土组成。(consist of)

_____

5. 中医理论知识有助于提升整体健康。(strengthen)

_____

Listening & Speaking

Task 1   Michael, a medical student, is explaining to Lisa, how her friend Rachel got chickenpox. Listen to the conversation and decide whether the following statements are true (T) or false (F).

Listening &
Speaking
Task 1

Diseases

(　) 1. Lisa is suffering from chickenpox.

(　) 2. Diseases that cannot be spread from one person to another are called communicable diseases.

(　) 3. Chickenpox and common cold are diseases caused by viruses.

(　) 4. Agents like the bacteria, fungi, protozoa and the virus can spread by air, food, carriers, water and direct contact.

(　) 5. We can get vaccinated only in the form of injection.

📖 **Notes**

1. …diseases can be of two types: communicable and non-communicable.

医药大学堂
WWW.YIYAODXT.COM

……疾病可分为两类：传染性和非传染性。

2. Communicable diseases are caused by agents like the bacteria, fungi, protozoa and the virus.

传染病是由细菌、真菌、原生动物和病毒等病原体引起的。

3. Viruses cause diseases like AIDS, chickenpox and common cold.

病毒会引起艾滋病、水痘和普通感冒等疾病。

4. The tuberculosis, chickenpox and common cold can be spread through air.

肺结核、水痘和普通感冒可以通过空气传播。

5. Another way is to get vaccinated in the form of injection or oral drops.

另一种方法是通过注射或滴剂接种疫苗。

"get/be vaccinated" 接种疫苗。

e. g. Should people continue to be vaccinated against seasonal influenza?

人们应该继续接种抵抗季节流感吗？

Listening &
Speaking
Task 2

Task 2 Lisa is not sleeping well, and feels tired, she goes to Hardy L. Ac. They are talking about the difference between Western and Eastern Medicine. Listen to the conversation and choose the best answer to each question you hear.

Western and Eastern Medicine

(　) 1. What do we know about Hardy from the conversation?

  A. He is the patient　　　　　　B. He is a licensed acupuncturist

  C. He is ageneral practice physician　　D. He is a friend of Lisa

(　) 2. What's the matter with Lisa?

  1. She is not sleeping well

  2. She has been tired

  3. She hasn't visited ageneral practice physician

  4. Both A and B

(　) 3. According to Hardy L. Ac, what is the main cause of Lisa's problem?

  A. She drinks too much alcohol　　B. She stays up too late

  C. Her job loss is a main cause　　　D. She takes too much junk food

(　) 4. What kind of health problem does "insomnia" belong to?

  A. Mental health problem

  B. Physical health problem

  C. Both mental and physical health problem

  D. Not mentioned

(　) 5. What's the difference between Western and Eastern Medicine?

  A. Western Medicine takes a holistic approach to medicine

  B. Eastern Medicine takes a reductionist approach

  C. Eastern medicine views the human body as a machine

  D. Eastern Medicine evaluates the entire person and seeks to heal the imbalances in the body

📖 **Notes**

1. L. Ac: licensed acupuncturist　注册针灸师。

2. I'll book you for regular acupuncture treatments to treat insomnia and stress.

我给你预订定期的针灸治疗来治疗失眠和压力。

3. It seems that you take a holistic approach to medicine, while my previous physician took a reductionist approach.

你采取的似乎是整体医学方法，而我之前的医生采取的是简化医学方法。

Task 3　**We should combine Traditional Chinese Medicine (TCM) and Western Medicine for maximum treatment benefits. Listen to the following passage and fill in the blanks with what you hear.**

Listening & Speaking Task 3

The _____1_____ of Traditional Chinese Medicine (TCM) and Western Medicine has been a highlight of China's _____2_____ and _____3_____ of the novel coronavirus disease (COVID-19). It was a significant guarantee for the current success the country has _____4_____ in the epidemic control, as well as a Chinese _____5_____ to share with the international community.

Task 4　**Work in groups, try to discuss the topic of "Diseases" and "Western and Eastern Medicine". Practice making the conversations with your partner according to what you hear in the Listening part.**

Partner A	Partner B
Greet!	Greet and ask diseases.
Introduce diseases.	Ask the type of disease of insomnia.
Explain the type.	Ask how to choose, western medicine or TCM.
Tell the difference between them.	Ask how to treat insomnia.
Regular acupuncture treatments can be applied.	Show the appreciation.

Reading B

Western Medicine

Western Medicine is based on clinical research and methods, including surgery as a treatment option. It encompasses all types of conventional medical treatment, including surgery, chemotherapy, radiation, and physical therapy. The majority of people in the United States receive most of their health care from doctors, nurses, physician's assistants (PAs) and other medical providers who practice in a medical

医药大学堂
WWW.YIYAODXT.COM

setting like a hospital, medical clinic, or doctor's office. This system is what most people think of when they hear the term "health care". It is usually referred to as "Western Medicine", also known as "allopathic", "conventional", or "traditional" medicine. This is the most common form of health care in the United States and the western world.

Western Medicine excels in the areas of testing and diagnostics. Most individuals in this country who are living with a chronic health condition received their diagnosis from a doctor practicing western medicine. The goal of western medical doctors in treating people with long-term disease or condition is to:

· Diagnose the disease

· Stop disease progression

· Relieve the symptoms associated with the disease

· Prevent the spread of the disease

· Cure the disease (if a cure is available)

· Improve quality of life

Western Medicine is Evidence-based

Western physicians make decisions about which treatment will be most helpful to their patients based on controlled, scientific studies. This approach is known as evidence-based medicine. Evidence-based treatment plans may include prescription medication, surgery, infusions, and other conventional procedures and therapies. Understanding the connection between lifestyle and physical health, western medicine practitioners are also more commonly encouraging lifestyle modifications——especially diet and exercise——for many Americans burdened by chronic health conditions.

What determines whether a treatment is evidence-based? Clinical trials are controlled research studies that are used to determine the efficacy and outcomes of treatment interventions, like drugs, new medical procedures, and even lifestyle changes. Clinical trials add to the medical knowledge related to disease prevention, diagnosis, and treatment. Clinical trials offer patients an opportunity to be treated with emerging, innovative therapies. In some cases, patients benefit greatly from their inclusion of clinical trials. However, clinical trials always pose a risk of harm to the participant, and clinical trial outcomes, like a new FDA-approved drug, usually benefit future patients. Participating in a clinical trial is a decision that should be taken seriously and discussed with your doctor and other trusted members of your health care and support teams.

Western Medicine: Labs and Diagnostics

Western medicine doctors play a key role in monitoring and assessing disease state and progression by using diagnostics, such as laboratory tests and imaging scans. These tests are vitally important, as they provide objective, biological data on changes in disease state. Results of these diagnostic tests may help you to understand what is working (and what isn't) in your health care plan and contribute to

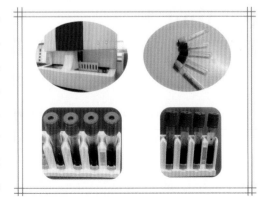

informed decision-making on both your and your provider's parts. Keep in mind that doctors can't and shouldn't order every test in the book to monitor a specific disease, and different doctors may opt to order different tests. Therefore, if there are specific tests you think you should receive based on your research, it's important to inquire about them with your doctor, rather than assuming they have already been performed or that they are even appropriate. Always maintain a record of your lab results.

(587 words)

Words and Expressions

encompass	/inˈkʌmpəs/	vt.	包含；包围
conventional	/kənˈvenʃənl/	adj.	符合习俗的，传统的
chemotherapy	/ˌkiːməʊˈθerəpi/	n.	[临床] 化学疗法
radiation	/ˌreidiˈeiʃn/	n.	辐射；放射物
allopathic	/ˌæləʊˈpæθik/	adj.	对抗疗法的
diagnostics	/ˌdaiəgˈnɒstiks/	n.	诊断学（用作单数）
chronic	/ˈkrɒnik/	adj.	慢性的
medication	/ˌmediˈkeiʃn/	n.	药物；药物治疗
infusion	/inˈfjuːʒn/	n.	输液；灌输
modification	/ˌmɒdifiˈkeiʃn/	n.	修改，修正
trial	/ˈtraiəl/	n.	试验；审讯
efficacy	/ˈefikəsi/	n.	功效，效力
emerging	/iˈmɜːrdʒiŋ/	adj.	新兴的；走向成熟的
innovative	/ˈinəveitiv/	adj.	革新的，创新的
assess	/əˈses/	vt.	评定；估价
opt	/ɒpt/	vi.	选择

After-reading Exercises

Task 1　Read the passage and choose the correct answer to each question.

(　) 1. Conventional medical treatment of western medicine includes _____ .

　　　A. chemotherapy　　　　　　　　B. radiation

　　　C. physical therapy　　　　　　　D. all of the above

(　) 2. Which of the following is Not referred to as "Western Medicine"?

　　　A. Allopathic medicine　　　　　　B. Traditional Chinese Medicine

　　　C. Conventional medicine　　　　　D. Traditional medicine

(　) 3. The goal of western medical doctors in treating patients is Not to _____ .

　　　A. seek to heal any imbalances in the body

　　　B. diagnose the disease

　　　C. oversee the medications given to patients

　　　D. diagnose the patients

(　) 4. According to the passage which of the following statements about "clinical trials" is correct?

A. Patients cannot benefit from their participating in clinical trials

B. Patients can benefit from their participating in clinical trials, as clinical trials are always safe to the participant

C. Patients can benefit from their participating in clinical trials, although clinical trials may pose a risk of harm to the participant

D. Patients can benefit from their participating in clinical trials, so we can take part in clinical trials without a second thought

(　　) 5. Laboratory tests and imaging scans are vitally important, because results of these tests _____ .

A. may help you to understand what is working (and what isn't) in your health care plan

B. contribute to informed decision-making on your parts

C. contribute to informed decision-making on your doctor's parts

D. all of the above

Task 2　Translate the following sentences into Chinese.

1. Western medicine is based on clinical research and methods, including surgery as a treatment option.

_____

2. Most individuals in this country who are living with a chronic health condition received their diagnosis from a doctor practicing western medicine.

_____

3. Evidence-based treatment plans may include prescription medication, surgery, infusions, and other conventional procedures and therapies.

_____

4. Clinical trials are controlled research studies that are used to determine the efficacy and outcomes of treatment interventions, like drugs, new medical procedures, and even lifestyle changes.

_____

5. Therefore, if there are specific tests you think you should receive based on your research, it's important to inquire about them with your doctor, rather than assuming they have already been performed or that they are even appropriate.

_____

Practical Writing

Job Posting

招聘广告主要指用来公布招聘信息的广告，要为应聘者提供一个获得更多信息的来源。人才招聘广告是企业员工招聘的重要工具之一。

招聘广告：a job posting，英文中也称为 a job advertisement，job ad，或 wanted ad。

Sample

Job Posting

Pharmacist

Tired of working in a hospital? Come work at Healthylife Pharm where you can make a difference！

The Company：

Healthylife Pharm is a progressive healthcare provider integrating community, hospital and compounding services.

The Position：

We are presently seeking an enthusiastic, experienced, self-motivated licensed pharmacist with a background in community pharmacy to join a dynamic team in our busy pharmacy. You will also be outgoing and team oriented.

Salary is $100,000 or more per year.

Requirements：

· Tertiary qualifications in pharmacy.

· Proficiency with Microsoft Word and Excel.

WHY SHOULD YOU APPLY?

· Top benefits.

· Excellent growth and advancement opportunities.

If you have the skillset described above, and are ready to take on a new and exciting challenge, then please email your application to：

healthylifepharm@email.com

招聘广告通常包含以下项目：

企业简介：The Company；

岗位与需求：The Position；Requirements；

应聘本岗位的理由：WHY SHOULD YOU APPLY？

联系方式：Contact us，等。

Task Sun Health Medical is going to employ some pharmacists. Please design a job posting for it with the information given below in Chinese.

药剂师招聘广告

企业简介：

向阳诊所位于福州工业园区，成立于 2007 年。我们一直致力于为福州本地和外籍人士提供国际化的医疗服务。

岗位需求：

我们正在寻找一个热情，经验丰富，自我激励的执业药师，有医院药学背景，加入我们充满活力的团队。性格外向，有团队精神。月薪 4000～6000 元。

要求应聘者具有大专及以上学历，具有药士或药师证；熟悉操作办公软件 Word、Excel。

有医院药房相关工作经验优先；英语口语熟练者待遇更优。

应聘本岗位的理由：

效益好，有良好的成长和提升机会。

如果你具备上述技能，并准备好接受新的、令人兴奋的挑战，请把您的申请发到诊所邮箱：
sunhealthmedical@ email. com

Job Posting

Pharmacist

Tired of working in a hospital? Come work at _____where you can make a difference!

_____ :

Sun Health Medical, _____

_____

_____ .

_____ :

_____

_____

You will also be outgoing and team oriented.

Salary _____ .

Requirements：

· _____ .

· Proficiency with Microsoft Word and Excel.

Those with _____ are preferred, _____

_____

_____ :

· Top benefits.

· Excellent growth and advancement opportunities.

If you have the skillset described above, and are ready to take on a new and exciting challenge, then please _____ to：

sunhealthmedical@ email. com

Grammar Tips

词类是指按照词在结构中能起的作用，即词的句法功能分的类。语言里有许许多多的词，它们是构造句子的"建筑材料"。英语单词根据词义及在句子中的作用划分为以下 12 类。

Parts of Speech

词类	缩略	意义	分类与例词	
名词 Noun	n.	名词表示人、物、地点等具体的名称，也可以指抽象概念的名称	专有名词：Beijing，China，Mary，the United States	
			普通名词：tree，family，love，air	
代词 Pronoun	pron.	代词就是用一个词代替别的词	人称代词：I，we，he，me，him，us	
			物主代词：my，your，our，mine，yours，ours	
			反身代词：myself，yourself，ourselves	
			指示代词：this，that，these，such，it，these	
			关系代词：who，which，that，whom	
			疑问代词：who，what，which	
			连接代词：who，what，which，whose	
			不定代词：some，any，nothing，a few	
形容词 Adjective	adj.	用于描述名词的外形、质地、性质、特征等	tall，short，fat，big，good，better，best	
副词 Adverb	adv.	描述动作发生的时间、地点、强弱等	now，then，here，slowly，late	
动词 Verb	v.	一般用来表示动作或状态的的词汇	实义动词：give，come，rise，run	
			系动词：get，become，turn，keep，seem	
			助动词：be，do，have，will，shall	
			情态动词：can，may，must	
数词 Numeral	num.	指表示数目多少或顺序多少的词	ten，tenth，two，second，one-third	
冠词 Article	art.	是一种虚词，只能与名词放在一起	a，an，the	
介词 Preposition	prep.	表示名词、代词等与句中其它词的关系	to，in，on，of，from，at	
连词 Conjunction	conj.	用于连接词与词，短语与短语，句与句	and，but，who，after，so，for	
感叹词 Interjection	interj.	具有表达情感的作用	well，oh，wow，ouch	
疑问词 Interrogative	int.	用来构建疑问句的词语	疑问代词：who，what，which，whose	
			疑问副词：when，where，how，why	
量词 Quantifier	quant.	通常用来表示人、事物或动作的数量单位	a couple of，a drop of，a bunch of	

Task 1   Identify the Parts of Speech of each underlined italicspart in the following sentences.

1. Mary's *sister* dances *well*.   _____，_____

2. Tom is *looking for* his *book*.

＿＿＿＿＿, ＿＿＿＿＿

3. *His* fathering is working *at* the company.

＿＿＿＿＿, ＿＿＿＿＿

4. Think well *before* you *act*.

＿＿＿＿＿, ＿＿＿＿＿

5. *I* have bought this cap for *two* years.

＿＿＿＿＿, ＿＿＿＿＿

6. *Well*, I *didn't* think to see you here!

＿＿＿＿＿, ＿＿＿＿＿

7. *The* wallpaper and paint match *pretty* well.

＿＿＿＿＿, ＿＿＿＿＿

8. *Nothing* can live *without* water.

＿＿＿＿＿, ＿＿＿＿＿

9. He struck *a* match *and* lit his cigarette.

＿＿＿＿＿, ＿＿＿＿＿

10. *His* latest film doesn't match his *previous* ones.

＿＿＿＿＿, ＿＿＿＿＿

Task 2 Choose the best answer to complete each sentence according to the Parts of Speech.

(　　) 1. The ＿＿＿＿＿ is just around the corner and you won't miss it.

    A. bicycles' shop　　　　　　　B. bicycles shop

    C. bicycle shop　　　　　　　　D. bicycle's shop

(　　) 2. What we have done is far from ＿＿＿＿＿ .

    A. satisfactory　　　　　　　　B. satisfied

    C. satisfaction　　　　　　　　D. satisfy

(　　) 3. The bicycle you saw isn't ＿＿＿＿＿ . It belongs to ＿＿＿＿＿ .

    A. me, you　　　　　　　　　B. mine, hers

    C. hers, his　　　　　　　　　D. his, hers

(　　) 4. Some architectural designs are better than ＿＿＿＿＿ .

    A. others　　　　　　　　　　B. another

    C. the other　　　　　　　　　D. the rest

(　　) 5. Nancy is considered to be ＿＿＿＿＿ the other students in her class.

    A. less intelligent　　　　　　B. the most intelligent

    C. intelligent as well　　　　　D. as intelligent as

(　　) 6. Last night he studied English ＿＿＿＿＿ midnight.

    A. for　　　　　　　　　　　B. by

    C. to　　　　　　　　　　　　D. until

(　　) 7. This kind of material expands ＿＿＿＿＿ the temperature increasing.

    A. to　　　　　　　　　　　　B. for

    C. with　　　　　　　　　　　D. at

(　　) 8. Please hurry up, ＿＿＿＿＿ we'll be late.

    A. and　　　　　　　　　　　B. but

    C. or　　　　　　　　　　　　D. so

(　　) 9. Professor, would you slow down a bit, please? I can't ＿＿＿＿＿ you.

    A. keep up with　　　　　　　B. put up with

    C. make up to　　　　　　　　D. hold on to

(   ) 10.   ——Write to me when you get home.

        ——I _____ .

      A. must   B. will

      C. should   D. can

Supplementary Reading

Human Disease

Diseases can be classified in a number of ways, depending on the information needed by the doctor or scientist.

Epidemiology and Epidemic Diseases

One way to classify diseases is by the population groups they affect or the way they spread. This is called epidemiology, and it is a very important science. Public health officials use epidemiology to study and manage society's response to disease.

Epidemiologists try to predict how likely it is that one or more diseases will occur in an area where the population is affected by a common circumstance, such as untreated drinking water. These predictions are based on mathematical formulas that determine the chance, or probability, of an outcome given particular circumstances.

Epidemiologists are also concerned with epidemic diseases——that is, diseases that strike many persons or entire populations within a relatively short period. History has seen many devastating epidemics, from the plague in Europe during the Middle Ages, to the influenza pandemic (global epidemic) of 1918-1919, to the COVID-19 currently gripping most of the world. When a disease stubbornly remains in the same region year after year, it is called an endemic disease. Yellow fever, for instance, is endemic to tropical South America and Africa.

Acute and Chronic Disease

Diseases are generally defined as either acute or chronic. An acute disease has a quick onset; most run a relatively short course, during which symptoms may be mild or severe. The common cold is a relatively mild acute disease of fairly short duration. SARS, or severe acute respiratory syndrome, also has a quick onset; but SARS can rapidly become very serious, even fatal. A chronic disease has a slow onset and a long duration that can last for years. Rheumatoid arthritis is an example of a chronic ailment with a very long course. Some diseases, such as bronchitis, have both acute and chronic forms.

Infectious and Noninfectious Diseases

One of the most important ways of classifying diseases is to distinguish between infectious and noninfectious diseases. Infectious diseases are caused by living organisms such as bacteria, fungi, protozoans, viruses, and parasites. Whatever the causative agent may be, it survives in the "host" person—— in other words, it is infectious. If it can be passed on to another person, it is also communicable. Noninfectious diseases are not caused by a living organism; and because they are not passed from one person to another, they also are noncommunicable.

Organ System Diseases

Frequently, diseases are classified according to the organ or organ system that has been affected. There are diseases of the respiratory system (pneumonia), cardiovascular system (coronary artery disease), nervous system (multiple sclerosis), and endocrine system (diabetes mellitus), among many others.

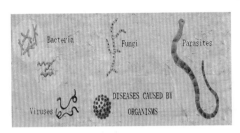

Localized and Systemic Diseases

Diseases and their associated signs and symptoms are further distinguished by the extent of their spread in the body. A local, or localized, ailment or symptom is confined to a particular site or single organ system, whereas a systemic disease affects the entire body. This is an important factor in treatment. For example, an infected cut may be treated with a topical antibiotic cream if the infection is limited to the site of the injury. If the infection invades deeper tissues and spreads to the bloodstream, the infectious organism can be carried to every organ in the body. To treat this, doctors must prescribe a systemic drug; this is usually an oral or injectable medication that can enter the bloodstream and fight the infection at all affected sites.

(581 words)

After-reading Exercises

Task   Decide whether the following statements are true (T) or false (F) according to the text.

( ) 1. The way to classify diseases by the population groups they affect or the way they spread is called epidemiology.

( ) 2. When a disease like yellow fever stubbornly remains in the same region year after year, it is called an epidemic disease.

( ) 3. An acute disease has a quick onset; most run a relatively short course, it can rapidly become very serious, even fatal.

( ) 4. Noninfectious diseases are caused by a living organism; and if they are not passed from one person to another, they also are noncommunicable.

( ) 5. To treat a systemic disease, doctors must prescribe an oral or injectable medication that can enter the bloodstream and fight the infection at all affected sites.

Vocabulary Tips

Root "herb"：来源于拉丁语 herba 草。

Example：herbal 药草的，草本植物的；herbicide 除草剂。

Prefix "ac-/acu-"：尖锐的。

Example：acupuncture 针灸，针刺疗法（-punct = prick 戳；扎）；acme 顶峰，顶点；acmesthesia针刺感觉；acute 急性的，敏锐的。

Suffix "-ology，-logy"：学问，科学。

Example：reflexology 反射学；反射疗法；biology：生物学。

Prefix "dia-"：通过，两者之间。

Example：diagnostic 诊断的，（-gno ＝know 知道）；diaphragm 横膈膜（-phragm ＝fence 围墙）。

Task　**Complete the sentences with the given words.**

biology	diagnostic	diaphragm	herbicide	acme

1. Doctor Smith wants to conduct at _____ examination of your liver.

2. In _____ class we had to dissect a frog.

3. The amount of toxic _____ now used on soy has public health implications.

4. His work is considered the _____ of cinematic art.

5. Professional singers use the air from their _____ to push out each note（音符）.

Proverbs and Sayings

◇Keep in good health through movement, and keep in good soul in the static.

养生在动，养心在静。

◇Diseases of the soul are more dangerous than those of the body.

心灵上的疾病比身体上的疾病更危险。

◇There are no such things as incurable; there are only things for which man has not found a cure.

没有什么不治之症，只有人类尚未发现其疗法之症。

题库

PPT

Unit **2**

Pharmacy and Pharmacist

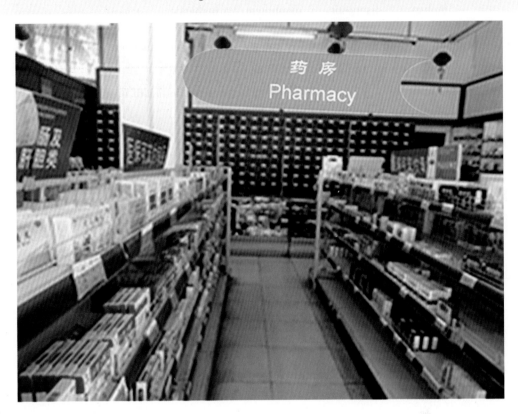

Unit Objectives

After studying this unit, you are expected to:

· master the vocabulary and technical terms related to pharmacy and pharmacist;

· understand the history of pharmaceutical development and the role of pharmacists;

· know English sentence components correctly.

And you should learn how to:

· communicate with others about the professional choice and future career prospects about pharmacy;

· write a registration form.

Introduction

医药大学堂
WWW.YIYAODXT.COM

Introduction

Pharmacy is the health science undertaking the discovery, production, control, disposal, safe and effective use of drugs. The scope of pharmacy practice includes more traditional roles such as compounding and dispensing of medications, and it also includes more modern services related to health care, including clinical services, reviewing medications for safety and efficacy, and providing drug information.

Pharmacists also known as chemists (Common wealth English) or druggists (North American), are health professionals who specialize in the use of medicines, as they deal with the composition, effects, mechanism of action and proper and effective use of drugs.

Warming-up

Task   Work in groups. Match the pictures to the proper statements. Then check your answers with your partner.

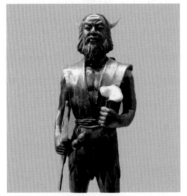

A

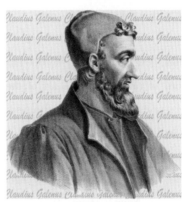

B

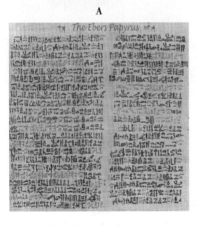

C

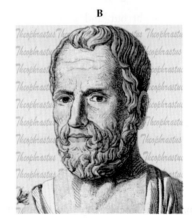

D

(　) 1. "The Ebers Papyrus" is an Egyptian medical papyrus of herbal knowledge and represents and best-preserved record of ancient Egyptian medicine known.

(　) 2. In Chinese mythology Shen Nong taught humans the use of the plow together with other aspects of basic agriculture, the use of medicinal plants.

(　) 3. The ancient Greek Theophrastus (371-286 B. C. E.) is known as the father of botany. He wrote two large books, *On the History of Plants* and *On the Causes of Plants*.

(　) 4. Galen, Greek physician, writer, and philosopher who exercised a dominant influence on medical theory and pharmacy.

Reading A

Pharmacy in Ancient Times

Before the Dawn of History

The development of Pharmacy parallels that of man. Ancient man learned from instinct, from observation of birds and beasts. Cool water, a leaf, dirt, or mud was his first soothing application. By trial, he learned which served him best. Eventually, he applied his knowledge for the benefit of others. Though these methods were crude, many of today's medicines spring from sources as simple and elementary as those which were within reach of early man.

Pharmacy in Ancient Babylonia

Babylon, jewel of ancient Mesopotamia, often called the cradle of civilization, provides the earliest known record of practice of the art of the apothecary. Practitioners of healing of this era (about 2600 B. C.) were priest, pharmacist and physician, all in one. Ancient Babylonian methods find counterpart in today's modern pharmaceutical, medical, and spiritual care of the sick.

Pharmacy in Ancient China

Chinese Pharmacy, according to legend, stems from Shen Nong (about 2000 B. C.), emperor who sought out and investigated the medicinal value of several hundred herbs. He is reputed to have tested many of them on himself, and to have written the first *Pen T-Sao*, or native herbal, recording 365 drugs. Still worshiped by native Chinese drug guilds as their patron god, Shen Nong conceivably examined many herbs, barks, and roots 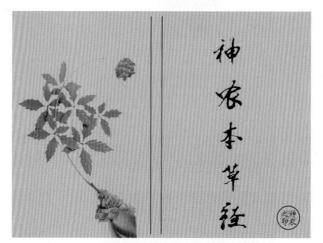 brought in from the fields, swamps, and woods that are still recognized in pharmacy today.

Days of the *Papyrus Ebers*

Though Egyptian medicine dates from about 2900 B. C. , best known and most important pharmaceutical record is the "Papyrus Ebers" (1500 B. C.), a collection of 800 prescriptions, mentioning 700 drugs. Pharmacy in ancient Egypt was conducted by two or more echelons: gatherers and preparers of drugs, and "chiefs of fabrication", or head pharmacists. They are thought to have worked in the "House of Life". The "Papyrus Ebers" might have been dictated to a scribe by a head pharmacist as he directed compounding activities in the drug room.

Theophrastus——Father of Botany

Theophrastus (about 300 B. C.), among the greatest early Greek philosophers and natural scientists, is called the "father of botany". He described over 500 plant species and devised an advanced classification scheme for plants. His observations and writings dealing with the medical qualities and peculiarities of herbs are unusually accurate, even in the light of present knowledge.

Galen——Experimenter in Drug Compounding

Of the men of ancient times whose names are known and revered among both the professions of Pharmacy and Medicine, Galen, undoubtedly, is the foremost. Galen（129-210 A. D.）practiced and taught both Pharmacy and Medicine in Rome; his principles of preparing and compounding medicines ruled in the Western world for 1,500 years; and his name still is associated with that class of pharmaceuticals compounded by mechanical means——galenicals. He was the originator of the formula for a cold cream, essentially similar to that known today. Many procedures Galen originated have their counterparts in today's modern compounding laboratories.

（483 words）

Reading A
Words and
Expressions

Words and Expressions			
pharmacy	/ˈfɑːməsi/	n.	药房；配药学，药剂学
pharmacist	/ˈfɑːməsist/	n.	药剂师
parallel	/ˈpærəlel/	vt.	使……与……平行
instinct	/ˈinstiŋkt/	n.	本能，直觉；天性
soothing	/ˈsuːðiŋ/	adj.	抚慰的；使人宽心的
application	/ˌæpliˈkeiʃn/	n.	应用；申请
eventually	/iˈventʃuəli/	adv.	最后，终于
elementary	/ˌeliˈmentri/	adj.	基本的；初级的
civilization	/ˌsivəlaiˈzeiʃn/	n.	文明；文化
apothecary	/əˈpɒθəkəri/	n.	药剂师；药师；药材商
priest	/priːst/	n.	牧师；神父
physician	/fiˈziʃn/	n.	医师，内科医师
counterpart	/ˈkaʊntəpɑːt/	n.	配对物；极相似的人或物
pharmaceutical	/ˌfɑːməˈsuːtikl/	adj.	制药（学）的
		n.	药物
legend	/ˈledʒənd/	n.	传奇；传说；说明
worship	/ˈwɜːʃip/	vt.	崇拜；尊敬
guild	/gild/	n.	协会，行会
conceivably	/kənˈsiːvəbli/	adv.	可以想象的是
bark	/bɑːk/	n.	树皮
swamp	/swɒmp/	n.	沼泽
prescription	/priˈskripʃn/	n.	药方；指示
echelon	/ˈeʃəlɒn/	n.	等级；阶层
fabrication	/ˌfæbriˈkeiʃn/	n.	制造，建造
dictate	/dikˈteit/	vt.	命令；口述
scribe	/skraib/	vt.	写下，记下
compound	/ˈkɒmpaʊnd/	v.	合成；混合

医药大学堂
WWW.YIYAODXT.COM

续表

philosopher	/fəˈlɒsəfə(r)/	n.	哲学家
botany	/ˈbɒtəni/	n.	植物学
revere	/rɪˈvɪə(r)/	vt.	敬畏；尊敬；崇敬
galenical	/gəˈlenɪk(ə)l/	n.	天然制剂；盖仑制剂
formula	/ˈfɔːmjələ/	n.	配方；准则

Proper Names

Babylonia	巴比伦王国，亚洲西南部的古代奴隶制国家，首都巴比伦（Babylon）
Mesopotamia	美索不达米亚（亚洲西南部）
Shen Nong	炎帝，号神农氏
Pen T-Sao	《本草经》又称《神农本草经》或《本经》，是中医四大经典著作之一，是已知最早的中药学著作
The Ebers Papyrus	《爱柏氏纸草纪事》，古埃及人编纂的一本有关药用植物书籍
Theophrastus	泰奥弗拉斯托斯，古希腊哲学家、自然科学家，"植物学之父"
Galen	盖伦，古罗马时代最著名医学家、动物解剖学家和哲学家

📖 Notes

1. Though these methods were crude, many of today's medicines spring from sources as simple and elementary as those which were within reach of early man.

虽然这些方法都很粗糙，但今天的许多药物都源于早期人类所能接触到的简单的基本的药材。

"those"指"those sources"，主句中which引导的定语从句修饰those。

e. g. He idled away his youth which he should have spent in learning.

他的青春年华本应该用于增长才干，而他却虚度过去了。

2. …the art of the apothecary; …pharmacist and physician, …

"Pharmacist" is a healthcare professional who practices in pharmacy. "Apothecary" is a historical name for a medical professional now called a pharmacist.

Pharmacist 药剂师（现代）；Apothecary 古字称的药剂师。

3. He is reputed to have tested many of them on himself, and to have written the first Pen T-Sao, or native herbal, recording 365 drugs.

中国世代传颂神农尝百草并著书《本草经》的故事。《本草经》记载了365种草药。

"be reputed to"意为"普遍认为，号称"。

e. g. He is reputed to be the best heart surgeon in the country.

他号称是这个国家最好的心脏外科医生。

"recording 365 drugs"为动词现在分词短语，相当于定语从句"which records 365 drugs"。

e. g. We have viewed the video recording of the incident.

我们已观看了该事件的录像。

4. Still worshiped by native Chinese drug guilds as their patron god …that are still recognized in pharmacy today.

神农从田野、沼泽和树林中采集了许多草药、树皮和根茎并验证其药理功能，当今的药学还认可这些发现，因此神农被中国的中药行会视为守护神。

"worshiped by…"过去分词短语在句子作结果状语。

e. g. The cup fell down to the ground, broken.

茶杯掉到了地上，破碎了。

5. ···best known and most important pharmaceutical record is the "Papyrus Ebers" (1500 B. C.) , a collection of 800 prescriptions, mentioning 700 drugs.

公元前 1500 年的《爱柏氏纸草纪事》是最著名、最重要的药用书籍，书中收集 800 个处方，记载 700 种药物。

"a collection of 800 prescriptions" 为 "Papyrus Ebers" 的同位语。

"mentioning 700 drugs" 现在分词短语作定语，相当于定语从句 "which mentions 700 drugs"。

6. Many procedures Galen originated have their counterparts in today's modern compounding laboratories.
盖伦发明的许多制药方法在当今现代配药实验室中也还有沿用。

"Many procedures Galen originated" 应为 "Many procedures (which/that) Galen originated" 为定语从句，省略关系代词 "which 或 that"。

After-reading Exercises

Task 1　Answer the following questions according to the text.

1. Do you know how the ancient men developed medicine before the dawn of history?

_____

2. Can you tell the contribution ancient Babylonian made to modern medicine?

_____

3. Why is Shen Nong still worshiped by native Chinese drug guilds as their patron god?

_____

4. Who is called the "father of botany"?

_____

5. What does "galenicals" refer to according to the passage?

_____

Task 2　Match the words (1-10) to the Chinese meanings (a-j) .

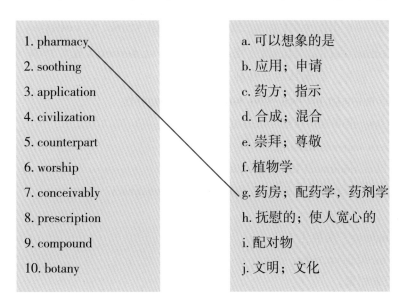

1. pharmacy
2. soothing
3. application
4. civilization
5. counterpart
6. worship
7. conceivably
8. prescription
9. compound
10. botany

a. 可以想象的是
b. 应用；申请
c. 药方；指示
d. 合成；混合
e. 崇拜；尊敬
f. 植物学
g. 药房；配药学，药剂学
h. 抚慰的；使人宽心的
i. 配对物
j. 文明；文化

Task 3   Fill in each blank with the proper form of the word or phrase given in brackets.

1. The doctor may _____ you something for that cough. (prescription)

2. Shortages of medicines, equipment and staff at health facilities throughout the country are _____ the health challenges. (compound)

3. We had to wait for the _____ to make up her prescription. (pharmacy)

4. Honey may _____ and control the cough for children. (soothing)

5. So is wheat, which is corn's _____ as the starch source of choice in the EU. (counterpart)

Task 4   Translate the following sentences into English using the words or phrases you have learned in this unit.

1. 古人本能地通过观察鸟兽进行学习。(learn from)

_____

2. 巴比伦为世界提供了已知最早的关于药师实践的记录。(provide)

_____

3. 根据传说，中国的药学起源于神农。(stem from)

_____

4. 他描述了 500 多种植物，并设计了一套先进的植物分类方案。(describe)

_____

5. 他的药物制备和复方原则统治了西方世界 1500 年。(rule)

_____

Listening & Speaking

Listening & Speaking Task 1

Task 1   Ajay, Peter, Akinyi and Jana are exchange students. Now they are talking about the different programs they will study at college. Listen to the conversation and decide whether the following statements are true (T) or false (F).

What's Your Major?

(   ) 1. These four students come from foreign countries.

(   ) 2. They are all in any of the same classes.

(   ) 3. Akinyi's major is nursing.

(   ) 4. Lee likes traditional Chinese culture.

(   ) 5. Jana will be a pharmacist, as she is studying pharmacy.

📖 **Notes**

1. exchange students   交换生。

2. Thanks for meeting up today.

感谢大家今天来相聚。

"meet up" means to meet a person or people in order to do something together   为了某种目的相见。

医药大学堂
WWW.YIYAODXT.COM

e. g. Let's meet up again. Can you manage next week sometime?

我们再见一次面吧。下周找个时间，行吗？

3. Yeah, we're all in the same boat.

我们将同舟共济。

To be in the same boat means to be in the same situation as others.

4. And my major is clinical medicine.

我的专业是临床医学。

Task 2　The four exchange students are talking about the reasons why Jana wants to be apharmacist. Listen to the conversation and choose the best answer to each question you hear.

Listening &
Speaking
Task 2

Why Do You Want to Be a Pharmacist?

(　　) 1. Why does Jana want to be a pharmacist?

        A. Hereally likes the sciences   B. Hereally likes helping people

        C. Both A and B   D. Not mentioned

(　　) 2. Which subject may be a plus in the study of pharmacy?

        A. English   B. Chemistry

        C. Nursing   D. Music

(　　) 3. What kind of role do pharmacists play between patients and medications?

        A. The first line between patients and medications

        B. The middle line between patients and medications

        C. The third line between patients and medications

        D. The last line between patients and medications

(　　) 4. Where does a pharmacist work?

        A. He can work at the hospital

        B. He can work at community pharmacy

        C. He can work at in a pharmaceutical company

        D. All are true

(　　) 5. Decide the following statements, which one is correct?

        A. Apharmacist should communicate effectively with a patient

        B. Jana likes to communicate with a patient

        C. Apharmacist is not a part of a health care team

        D. Jana doesn't like to be a pharmacist

📖 Notes

1. Walgreens　沃尔格林，美国最大连锁药店。

2. I think pharmacist should also be competent to communicate effectively with a patient.

我想药剂师也应该能与病人进行有效的沟通。

"be competent to do"：能胜任的，擅长于……

e. g. My major and working experience will enable me to be competent forthis position.

我所学的专业和已有的工作经验使我有能力胜任这份工作。

医药大学堂
WWW.YIYAODXT.COM

Task 3 The use of prescription is common in our life. Listen to the following passage and fill in the blanks with what you hear.

Whenever a doctor writes a prescription for a drug or treatment, a _____1_____ is the person who _____2_____ out the medication and makes sure a patient knows how to take it safely. And while _____3_____ a prescription often means a visit to the local drug store or grocery store, pharmacists also work in _____4_____. Typically, pharmacists spend most of the day standing at a counter, preparing and dispensing medication. They may also personalize or "_____5_____" the medication, though that is now less common than it used to be.

Task 4 Work in groups, try to discuss the topic of "What's your major?" and "Why do you choose this major?" Practice making the conversations with your partner according to what you hear in the Listening part.

Partner A	Partner B
Greet.	Greet and ask the major.
Introduce the major.	Ask the reason for choice.
Explain and express the deep love for major.	Ask the place of work.
Tell the places a pharmacist may work in.	Ask the importance of the job.
Tell importance of the job.	Express best wishes.

Reading B

Pharmacists

Pharmacists dispense prescription medications to patients and offer expertise in the safe use of prescriptions. They also may conduct health and wellness screenings, provide immunizations, oversee the medications given to patients, and provide advice on healthy lifestyles.

Types of Pharmacists

Community pharmacists work in retail stores such as chain drug stores or independently owned pharmacies. They dispense medications to patients and answer any questions that patients may have about prescriptions, over-the-counter medications, or any health concerns that the patient may have. They also may provide some primary care services such as giving flu shots.

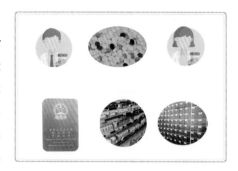

Clinical pharmacists work in hospitals, clinics, and other healthcare settings. They spend little time dispensing prescriptions. Instead, they are involved in direct patient care. Clinical pharmacists may go on rounds in a hospital with a physician or healthcare team. They recommend medications to give to patients and oversee the dosage and timing of the delivery of those medications. They also may conduct some medical tests and offer advice to patients. For example, pharmacists working in a diabetes clinic may counsel patients on how and when to take medications, suggest healthy food choices, and monitor patients' blood sugar.

Consultant pharmacists advise healthcare facilities or insurance providers on patient medication use or improving pharmacy services. They also may give advice directly to patients, such as helping seniors manage their prescriptions.

Pharmaceutical industry pharmacists work in areas such as marketing, sales, or research and development. They may design or conduct clinical drug trials and help to develop new drugs. They may also help to establish safety regulations and ensure quality control for drugs.

Some pharmacists work as college professors. They may teach pharmacy students or conduct research.

Important Qualities for Pharmacists

Analytical skills. Pharmacists must provide safe medications efficiently. To do this, they must be able to evaluate a patient's needs and the prescriber's orders, and have extensive knowledge of the effects and appropriate circumstances for giving out a specific medication.

Communication skills. Pharmacists frequently offer advice to patients. They might need to explain how to take medicine, for example, and what its side effects are. They also need to offer clear direction to pharmacy technicians and interns.

Computer skills. Pharmacists need computer skills in order to use any electronic health record (EHR) systems that their organization has adopted.

Detail oriented. Pharmacists are responsible for ensuring the accuracy of the prescriptions they fill. They must be able to find the information that they need to make decisions about what medications are appropriate for each patient, because improper use of medication can pose serious health risks.

Managerial skills. Pharmacists——particularly those who run a retail pharmacy——must have good managerial skills, including the ability to manage inventory and oversee a staff.

Education for Pharmacists

Prospective pharmacists are required to have a Doctor of Pharmacy (Pharm. D.) degree. A Pharm. D. program includes courses in chemistry, pharmacology, and medical ethics. Students also complete supervised work experiences, sometimes referred to as internships, in different settings such as hospitals and retail pharmacies.

Some pharmacists who own their own pharmacy may choose to get a master's degree in business administration (MBA) in addition to their Pharm. D. Degree. Others may get a degree in public health.

Pharmacists also must take continuing education courses throughout their career to keep up with the latest advances in pharmacological science.

(549 words)

Words and Expressions

dispense	/dɪˈspens/	vt.	分配，分发
expertise	/ˌekspɜːˈtiːz/	n.	专门知识；专门技术
screening	/ˈskriːnɪŋ/	n.	筛查，筛检
immunization	/ˌɪmjunaɪˈzeɪʃn/	n.	免疫
oversee	/ˌəʊvəˈsiː/	vt.	监督；审查
over-the-counter	/ˌəʊvə ðə ˈkaʊntə(r)/	adj.	非处方的
dosage	/ˈdəʊsɪdʒ/	n.	剂量，用量
diabetes	/ˌdaɪəˈbiːtiːz/	n.	糖尿病；多尿症
counsel	/ˈkaʊnsl/	vt.	建议；劝告
		n.	法律顾问；忠告
insurance	/ɪnˈʃʊrəns/	n.	保险；保险费
analytical	/ˌænəˈlɪtɪkl/	adj.	分析的；解析的
intern	/ˈɪntɜːn/	n.	实习生，实习医师
inventory	/ˈɪnvəntri/	n.	存货，存货清单
pharmacology	/ˌfɑːməˈkɒlədʒi/	n.	药物学，药理学
supervise	/ˈsuːpəvaɪz/	v.	监督；管理；指导
flu shot			流感疫苗；预防针

Proper Names

electronic health record (EHR)	电子健康档案，电子病历
Doctor of Pharmacy (Pharm. D.) degree	药学博士学位
medical ethics	医德；[基医] 医学伦理学
Master of Business Administration (MBA)	工商管理学硕士

After-reading Exercises

Task 1   Read the passage and choose the correct answer to each question.

(　) 1. According to the passage pharmacists may not _____ .

    A. conduct health and wellness screenings

    B. oversee the medications given to patients

    C. diagnose the patients

    D. provide advice on healthy lifestyles

(　) 2. Which of the following is not the main duty of Clinical pharmacists?

    A. Spend most of time dispensing prescriptions for patients

    B. Recommend medications to give to patients

    C. Oversee the dosage and timing of the delivery of those medications

    D. Conduct some medical tests and offer advice to patients

(   ) 3. Which type of pharmacists may design or conduct clinical drug trials and help to develop new drugs?

      A. Community pharmacists

      B. Clinical pharmacists

      C. Consultant pharmacists

      D. Pharmaceutical industry pharmacists

(   ) 4. Which skills are essential for pharmacists to offer advice to patients more efficiently?

      A. Analytical skills   B. Computer skills

      C. Communication skills   D. Managerial skills

(   ) 5. Some pharmacists who run their own pharmacy may _____ .

      A. get a master's degree in business administration (MBA)

      B. get Pharm. D. degree

      C. get a degree in public health only

      D. get both Pharm. D. degree and a master's degree in business administration (MBA)

Task 2   Translate the following sentences into Chinese.

1. Pharmacists also may conduct health and wellness screenings, provide immunizations, oversee the medications given to patients, and provide advice on healthy lifestyles.

_____

2. They dispense medications to patients and answer any questions that patients may have about prescriptions, over-the-counter medications, or any health concerns that the patient may have.

_____

3. They recommend medications to give to patients and oversee the dosage and timing of the delivery of those medications.

_____

4. To do this, they must be able to evaluate a patient's needs and the prescriber's orders, and have extensive knowledge of the effects and appropriate circumstances for giving out a specific medication.

_____

5. Pharmacists also must take continuing education courses throughout their career to keep up with the latest advances in pharmacological science.

_____

Practical Writing

Registration Forms

　　表格一般是事先印制好的、供填写文字或数字的书面材料。表格可以简明扼要地提供准确信息。可以说，填表是最基本的写作实践。表格的种类繁多，形式多样，用途十分广泛。申请入学、寻找工作、银行开户、出入境等都必须填写各类表格。

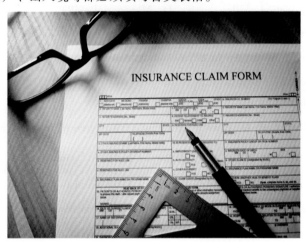

Sample

Registration Form for New Students

Full Name：Zhang Hua

Sex：Male

Date of Birth：June 20, 1996

Place of Birth：Nanjing, Jiangsu Province, China

Address：23 Xinhua Road, Jixi District, Nanjing, Jiangsu

Mobile Phone：18912345678

E-mail：zhanghua@163. com

School Attended：Nanjing NO. 1 Middle School

Hobbies：Swimming, Painting, Basketball

表格通常包含以下项目：

姓名：Name。

性别：Sex/Gender；男 Male（M）；女 Female（F）。

年龄：Age。

出生年月：Date of Birth，按日月年或月日年的顺序填写。

出生地或籍贯：Place of Birth。

婚姻状况：Marital Status；未婚：single/unmarried；已婚 married。

教育背景：Education Background，按照从近到远的时间顺序填写。

工作简历：Work Experience。

兴趣爱好：Hobbies。

证明人：Reference（s）。

Task   Liu Yang is going to visit Singapore. Fill in the Singapore Visa Application Form with his personal information given below in Chinese.

刘洋，生于 1995 年 6 月 6 日，男，未婚，中国籍，住中国上海南京路 50 号（出生地同上）。现为复旦大学医学院药学专业学生，去新加坡旅游，计划停留 5 天。申请日期 2019 年 8 月 17 日。

Singapore Visa Application Form

Full name _____   Chinese characters _____

Date and place of birth _____

Gender _____   Marital status _____

Nationality _____   Nationality at birth _____

Permanent address _____

Present address _____

Occupation _____

Reason for visit _____

Proposed duration of stay _____

Signature _____   Date _____

Grammar Tips

句子是按照一定的语法规律组成的，表达一个完整的意义。在句中起着不同语法作用的成分，叫做句子成分。一个句子一般由两部分构成，即主语和谓语部分，这两部分也叫做句子的主要成分。句子的次要成分包括宾语，定语，状语，表语等。

Sentence Components

句子成分	意义	充当词类
主语 Subject	句子要说明的人或物	一般在句首，由名词、主格代词、数词、动词不定式、动名词等具有名词性质的短语或句子充当
	e. g. Smoking does harm to the health.	
谓语 Predicate	说明主语的动作或状态	一般在主语之后，由动词构成，是英语时态语态变化的主角
	e. g. I bought the medicine in the shop yesterday.	

医药大学堂
WWW.YIYAODXT.COM

续表

句子成分	意义	充当词类
表语 Predicative	说明主语的性质、特征、状态身份	位于系动词后，可为名词、代词、动名词、形容词、副词、不定式等
	e. g. His wish is to become a pharmacist.	
宾语 Object	表示动作的承受对象	位于及物动词或介词后，由名词、宾格代词、数词、动词不定式、动名词等具有名词性质的词或短语充当
	e. g. I ate an apple this morning.	
定语 Attributive	修饰或限定名词或代词	置于名词或代词前后皆可，由名词、形容词、代词、数词、动名词、不定式、介词短语等构成
	e. g. The man on the right is my nurse.	
状语 Adverbial	修饰形容词、副词、动词或整个句子	可做状语的词多为副词、不定式、介词短语、分词短语等具有副词性质的词、短语或句子
	e. g. We'll go where the patient need us.	
补语 Complement	补充说明主语或宾语	可由形容词、名词、代词、数词或介词短语等充当
	e. g. We call him the doctor.	
同位语 Appositive	对前面的名词或代词作进一步的解释	通常由名词、形容词、数词、代词或从句充当
	e. g. There was little hope that they would survive.	
插入语 Parenthesis	对一句话做附加解释	通常由形容词、副词、介词短语、动词不定式、现在分词或从句充当
	e. g. This, I think, is the best way to help them.	

Task 1 Identify the Sentence Component of each underlined italics part in the following sentences.

1. The *students* got on *the school* bus.   _____, _____

2. I *shall answer* your question *after class*.   _____, _____

3. *His* job is *to train swimmers*.   _____, _____

4. He took many *photos* of the palaces *in Beijing*.   _____, _____

5. There *is going to* be *an American film* tonight.   _____, _____

6. *His wish* is *to become a scientist*.   _____, _____

7. He *managed to* finish *the work* in time.   _____, _____

8. Do you have *anything else to say*?   _____, _____

9. *To be honest*, your pronunciation is *not* so good.   _____, _____

10. *It* is *our duty* to keep our classroom *clean and tidy*. _____, _____, _____

Task 2 Choose the best answer to complete each sentence according to the Sentence Component.

(　　) 1. _____ in English in class every day is important.

　　　A. Speak   B. Talking

　　　C. Saying   D. To tell

(　) 2. The doctor as well as the nurses _____ great concern for the patients.

    A. show　　　　　　　B. shows

    C. have shown　　　　D. are showing

(　) 3. The days are _____warmer and warmer in spring.

    A. getting　　　　　　B. looking

    C. seeming　　　　　　D. going

(　) 4. I don't know _____ .

    A. how to do　　　　　B. what to do

    C. where to do　　　　D. when to do

(　) 5. I saw him _____ basketball with Jack an hour ago.

    A. plays　　　　　　　B. to play

    C. played　　　　　　D. playing

(　) 6. We all know _____ our duty to clean our classroom after school every day.

    A. that　　　　　　　B. this

    C. which　　　　　　　D. it

(　) 7. Children _____ a happy life in China.

    A. lead　　　　　　　B. living

    C. has　　　　　　　　D. leading

(　) 8. Do you have anything _____?

    A. saying　　　　　　B. to say

    C. said　　　　　　　D. say

(　) 9. You can see these signs in a hospital. _____ can you see them?

    A. Where else　　　　　B. Where place else

    C. Where else place　　D. Else where

(　) 10. _____, some railway workers are busy repairing the train.

    A. Them　　　　　　　B. He

    C. They　　　　　　　D. Theirs

Supplementary Reading

Hospital Pharmacist Role
Expands in Patient Care

Ken Krizner

May 23, 2019

Why hospital pharmacists are playing an increasingly large role in patient care and why their involvement can boost medication outcomes and reduce errors.

Hospital pharmacists are not unlike pharmacists in other practice settings. Their primary objective is to ensure that patients experience safe medication use.

Beyond that purpose, however, the role of hospital pharmacists (also known as health-system or clinical pharmacists) encompasses a broad range of duties with the ultimate goal of providing quality care during an inpatient stay, ensuring a seamless transition of care, and reducing the number of medication errors.

Hospital pharmacists consult on diagnosis, examine patient charts, and conduct patient evaluations to recommend a course of treatment, and choose the appropriate dosing of medications and evaluate their effectiveness.

"In health systems, pharmacists are more involved with direct patient care than ever before" says Norman Tomaka, a clinical consultant pharmacist in Melbourne, Florida. "There's an incredible opportunity for pharmacists to improve patient outcomes. I see that happening more and more."

With the continued trend toward value-based payment models, hospital pharmacists are taking an active part in efforts to reduce readmission rates.

"The role of pharmacists in the hospital is shifting from a distribution-centric model to more of a service delivery focus" says Eric Maroyka, Pharm. D, director of the Center on Pharmacy Practice Advancement section for the American Society of Health-System Pharmacists (ASHP). "They're part of an inter-professional team that may cut across different settings of care. Some of this is driven by a move to value-based care, such as CMS' quality measures and readmission targets."

How Health Systems Use Pharmacists to Reduce Readmissions

For patients with chronic conditions, hospital pharmacists can collaborate with physicians to manage disease states such as hypertension and chronic obstructive pulmonary disease, mainly through patient education and counselling, drug safety management, medication review, monitoring and reconciliation, detection and control of specific risk factors, and outcomes.

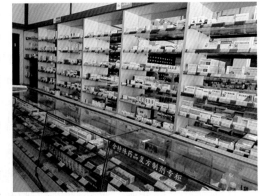

These examples of interactions show the value of the hospital pharmacist participating in rounds as part of the care team.

"Many times, the body stresses when someone is in the hospital" says Brook Des Rivieres, Pharm. D, MS, a member-spokeswoman for the American Pharmacists Association (APhA). "What works at home may not work in the hospital. Hospital pharmacists can make sure prescriptions and doses are clinically appropriate."

Des Rivieres describes the hospital pharmacist as a watchdog. "We're the safety net," she points out. "A provider may order a drug therapy, but it may not be administered until the pharmacist does a safety check. That's the biggest contribution pharmacists make in the inpatient setting."

Fewer Medication Errors

Numerous studies show hospital pharmacists substantially contribute to safer medication use by collaborating with other providers, and they improve the quality (reduced medication discrepancies) of admission and discharge reconciliation by exercising oversight.

Further studies document that pharmacists identify a significantly higher number of medications taken per patient, including more over-the-counter and herbal medications, compared with nurses, and they contact patients' outpatient pharmacies significantly more often than nurses.

Fewer errors are found when a pharmacist, rather than a physician, completes a patient's medication reconciliation during a hospital stay, according to a study published in March 2016.

"There has been lots of research that documents the important role of hospital pharmacists," Boothe stresses.

(Ken Krizner is a freelance writer based in Cleveland, Ohio.)

(563 words)

After-reading Exercises

Task　Decide whether the following statements are true (T) or false (F) according to the text.

(　) 1. Hospital pharmacists are more important than pharmacists in other practice settings.

(　) 2. The ultimate goal of hospital pharmacists is to reduce the readmission rate of hospital patients.

(　) 3. Hospital pharmacists are involved in patient care as part of a care team.

(　) 4. For patients with high blood pressure and chronic obstructive pulmonary disease, hospital pharmacists can work with doctors to manage the disease status.

(　) 5. Hospital pharmacists can safely use medications on their own, without the need for collaboration with other providers.

Vocabulary Tips

Root "pharmaco-, pharmac-"：药学、药、药理、药物。

Example：pharmacy 药房，药剂学，制药业；pharmacology 药物学，药理学；pharmacist 药剂师；pharmacopoeia 药典；pharmaceutics 制药学，配药学。

Root "-scrib"：写。来源于拉丁动词 scribere（= to write）。

Example：prescribe 开处方，规定，命令；transcribe 抄写，（播放）录音，（播放）录像；describe 描述，描写。

Task　Complete the sentences with the given words.

pharmacist　Pharmacopoeia　describe　pharmacology　prescribe

1. As a medical student 20 years ago, I learned all about anatomy, physiology and _____.

2. The physician may _____ but not administer the drug.

3. We had to wait for the _____ to make up her prescription.

4. The revised monograph for the new ORS（补液盐）formula will be published in the fourth edition of the International _____.

5. His novels nicely _____ life in Britain between the wars.

Proverbs and Sayings

◇There is no safe medicine, only a safe pharmacist. Use what I have learned and do what I can.

没有安全的药物，只有安全的药师，用我所学，尽我所能。

◇As a doctor, he must not be greedy for fame and devote himself to rescue.

为医者，须绝驰骛利名之心，专博施救援之志。

◇Bitter pills may have wholesome effects.

良药苦口利百病。

题库

Unit **3**

Drug Classification

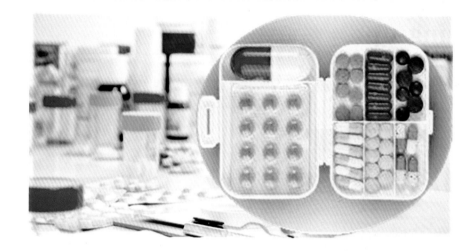

PPT

Unit Objectives

After studying this unit, you are expected to:

· master the vocabulary and technical terms related to classification of drugs;

· understand the general knowledge of drug classification, especially prescription and over-the-counter drugs;

· know English Simple Sentences correctly.

And you should learn how to:

· communicate with others about the differences and connections between Rx and OTC drugs;

· write a resume.

Introduction

Introduction

A drug class is a term used to describe medications that are grouped together because of their similarity. There are three dominant methods of classifying these groups:

· By their mechanism of action, meaning the specific biochemical reaction that occurs when you take a drug;

· By their physiologic effect, meaning the specific way in which the body responds to a drug;

· By their chemical structure.

As newer and more advanced drugs are being introduced into the market each year, the classification of drugs will likely become even more diverse and distinct, reflecting our ever-expanding knowledge about human biochemistry as a whole.

By noting the classification of a drug, you and your doctor can have a better understanding of what to expect when you take it, what the risks are, and which drugs you can switch to if needed. The aim of drug classification is to ensure that you use a drug safely to achieve the utmost benefit. Ultimately, every time you take a drug, your body chemistry is altered.

Warming-up

Task   Work in groups. Match the pictures to the proper statements.
Then check your answers with your partner.

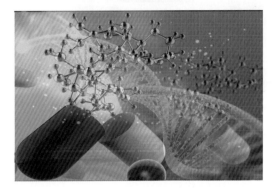

A

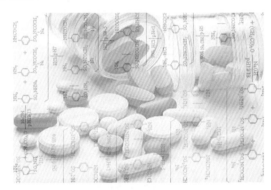

B

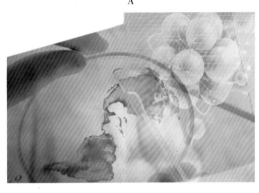

C

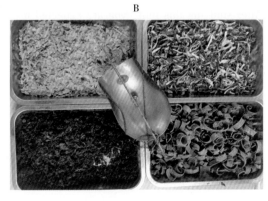

D

(　) 1. Natural drugs refer to animal drugs, plant drugs and mineral drugs that have been proved by the modern medical system to have certain pharmacological activities.

(　) 2. Chemical drugs refer to the active components extracted from natural minerals, plants and animals, as well as drugs that have been chemically synthesized or produced by biosynthesis.

(　) 3. Biological drugs are primary and secondary metabolites of an organism, including biological products, or a component of an organism, or even an entire organism, used as a medical agent for diagnosis and treatment.

(　) 4. Genetic engineering drugs, essentially proteins, are currently obtained mainly by microbial fermentation and animal cell culture.

Reading A

Prescription Drugs and Over-The-Counter Drugs：Do You Know the Difference？

Drugs are chemical substances which by interacting with the biological systems produce some changes in them. There are a variety of drugs available for use in the diagnosis, cure, treatment, or prevention of disease. These drugs fall into two broad categories：prescription drugs and over-the-counter（OTC）drugs.

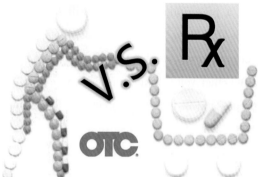

Prescription drugs and OTCs each have their place in improving the health and wellness of patients throughout the world. Understanding the difference between OTCs and prescription medications can help patients, at their local drug stores and businesses purchasing medications from drug wholesalers, make better decisions regarding their use.

In the U. S. , the Food and Drug Administration（FDA）determines which medications require a prescription to be dispensed by pharmacies. Several types of medical professionals can write prescriptions, including physicians, physician assistants, dentists, optometrists, nurse practitioners, psychiatrists, and some advanced practice nurses. Veterinarians can write prescriptions for animals only.

In China and many other countries, prescription drugs are medications that require a prescription, from a doctor or other medical professional authorized to write prescriptions, to be dispensed. Over-the-counter drugs are medications consumers can purchase without a prescription at drug stores, groceries, or other stores.

Key Differences

The biggest difference, of course, between prescription and over-the-counter drugs is that prescription medications require a doctor or other medical professional's authorization to obtain. Here are some of the other key differences between prescription and OTC drugs.

Prescription medications are specially tailored for use by a specific person for a specific use. OTC medications are considered safe for just about everyone and may have a variety of intended purposes. When doctors write prescriptions, they take into consideration a lot of information about their patients, including their current condition, other medications they may be taking, their vital statistics, and drug allergies they may have. That's why a prescription medication that is safe and effective for one person may be dangerous for another.

OTC drugs should only be used to treat minor ailments. Major illnesses and diseases require the use of more powerful prescription drugs and other medical treatments.

OTC drugs aren't as strong as prescription drugs, but they have a wider margin of safety. This means a wider range of people can safely use OTC drugs than can use the more specifically tailored prescription drugs.

OTC drugs typically have lower dosages than prescription drugs. There are quite a few prescription drugs that are available as OTC drugs because, when sold over-the-counter, the dosage is much lower than it is in the medication's prescription form.

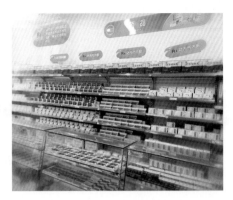

In general, OTC drugs are less expensive than prescription drugs. There are some generic prescription medications that are cheaper than OTC drugs, but, in most cases, a prescription medication will be far more expensive than an OTC drug. In the case of drugs used to treat cancer and other serious diseases, the cost of prescription drugs can be very expensive.

Whether you're taking prescription or non-prescription medication, it's important that you follow the directions and use the medication only for its intended purpose. Keeping up with expiration dates will also help you avoid taking ineffective drugs.

(519 words)

Reading A
Words and
Expressions

Words and Expressions			
substance	/ˈsʌbstəns/	n.	物质；实质；资产；主旨
interact	/ˌintərˈækt/	vt./vi.	互相影响；互相作用
biological	/ˌbaiəˈlɒdʒikl/	adj.	生物的；生物学的
diagnosis	/ˌdaiəgˈnəusis/	n.	诊断
category	/ˈkætəgəri/	n.	范畴；类别，种类
wellness	/ˈwelnəs/	n.	健康
medications	/ˌmediˈkeiʃn/	n.	药物；药物治疗（处理）
wholesaler	/ˈhəulseilə(r)/	n.	批发商
regarding	/riˈgɑːdiŋ/	prep.	关于；就……而论
optometrist	/ɒpˈtɒmətrist/	n.	验光师；视力测定者
practitioner	/prækˈtiʃənə(r)/	n.	开业者，从业者，执业医生
psychiatrist	/saiˈkaiətrist/	n.	精神病学家，精神病医生
veterinarian	/ˌvetəriˈneəriən/	n.	兽医
authorize	/ˈɔːθəraiz/	vt.	批准；授权给；委托代替
grocery	/ˈgrəusəri/	n.	食品杂货店；食品杂货
authorization	/ˌɔːθəraiˈzeiʃn/	n.	授权，认可；批准，委任
tailor	/ˈteilə(r)/	n.	裁缝
		v.	专门制作；调整；迎合
intended	/inˈtendid/	adj.	有意的；打算中的
vital	/ˈvaitl/	adj.	至关重要的；生死攸关的
allergy	/ˈælədʒi/	n.	过敏症；反感；厌恶
ailment	/ˈeilmənt/	n.	小病；不安
margin	/ˈmɑːdʒin/	n.	边缘；利润；页边的空白
generic	/dʒəˈnerik/	adj.	类的；一般的；非商标的

医药大学堂
WWW.YIYAODXT.COM

non-prescription	/ˌnɑːnprɪˈskrɪpʃn/	adj.	非处方的
expiration	/ˌekspəˈreɪʃn/	n.	呼气；终结；届期

Proper Names

prescription drugs		处方药，缩写 Rx，该符号源自拉丁语 Recipe "请取……" 的意思
over-the-counter drugs		非处方药，缩写 OTC
Food and Drug Administration（FDA）		美国食品和药物管理局
expiration date		药品的有效期，指药品在规定的贮藏条件下质量能够符合规定要求的期限

📖 **Notes**

1. These drugs fall into two broad categories.

这些药物分为两大类。

"fall into" 意为 "落入；分成"。

e. g. The problems generally fall into two categories.

这些问题一般属于两种类别。

2. Prescription drugs and OTCs each have their place in improving the health and wellness of patients throughout the world.

处方药和非处方药在改善世界各地患者的健康和保健方面各有其作用。

"have … place in" 意为 "有……地位在……"。

e. g. Sarcasm and demeaning remarks have no place in parenting.

挖苦和贬损的言语不应用来教育子女。

3. …, at their local drug stores and businesses purchasing medications from drug wholesalers, ……

在当地药店和从药品批发商那里购买药品，……

地点介词短语插入句中，前后逗号隔开。

4. Several types of medical professionals can write prescriptions, including physicians, physician assistants, dentists, optometrists, nurse practitioners, psychiatrists, and some advanced practice nurses.

几种类型的医疗专业人员可以开具处方，包括医生、医师助理、牙医、验光师、执业护士、精神病医生和一些高级执业护士。

5. The biggest difference, of course, between prescription and over-the-counter drugs is that prescription medications require a doctor or other medical professional's authorization to obtain.

当然，处方药和非处方药最大的区别在于，处方药需要医生或其他医疗专业人士的授权才能获得。

"of course" 意为 "一定，当然"，插入语成分，用在句中，前后逗号隔开。"that" 引导表语从句，不可省。

6. When doctors write prescriptions, they take into consideration a lot of information about their patients, including their current condition, other medications they may be taken, their vital statistics, and drug allergies they may have.

当医生开处方时，他们会考虑病人的很多信息，包括他们目前的状况，他们可能服用的其他药物，他们的生命数据，以及他们可能有的药物过敏。

"take into consideration/account" 意为 "顾及；考虑到……"

e. g. When buying an apartment, people usually take into account its price, position, surroundings and so on.

买房时，人们通常会考虑房子的价格、位置、环境等因素。

7. There are quite a few prescription drugs that are available as OTC drugs because, when sold over-the-counter, the dosage is much lower than it is in the medication's prescription form.

有相当多的处方药可以用作非处方药，因为在作非处方销售时，剂量要比在处方上的剂量低得多。

"that" 引导定语从句修饰限定 "a few prescription drugs"；"because" 引导原因状语从句；"when" 则引导时间状语从句补充原因状语。

After-reading Exercises

Task 1　Answer the following questions according to the text.

1. What does the drug do through this passage?

_____

2. What are prescription drugs and OTC drugs?

_____

3. Whocan write prescriptions in the U. S. ?

_____

4. Why do doctors take patient information into account when prescribing?

_____

5. Can you tell the differences between prescription and OTC drugs?

_____

Task 2　Match the following terms (1-10) to the Chinese meanings (a-j).

1. physician assistants	a. 执业护士
2. nurse practitioners	b. 当地药店
3. local drug stores	c. 药品批发商
4. medical professional	d. 非处方药
5. drug allergies	e. 有效期
6. drug wholesalers	f. 药物过敏
7. expiration dates	g. 医生助理
8. ineffective drugs	h. 医疗专业人士
9. OTC drugs	i. 无效药物
10. prescription drugs	j. 处方药

Task 3　Fill in each blank with the proper form of the word or phrase given in brackets.

1. The test is used _____ a variety of diseases. （diagnosis）

2. The controversy _____ vitamin C is unlikely to be resolved in the near future. （regard）

3. Prescription medications require a doctor's _____ to obtain. （authorize）

4. The experiment had the reverse effect to what was _____ . （intend）

5. One of the things we quickly found out when developing virtual spaces was that people want to know who they are _____ with. （interact）

Task 4　Translate the following sentences into English using the words or phrases you have learned in this unit.

1. 有各种各样的药物可用来诊断、治愈、治疗或预防疾病。（available）

_____

2. 非处方药被认为对几乎每个人都是安全的，可能有各种各样的预期目的。（consider；variety）

_____

3. 即使是开处方，也必须考虑到关于药物的文化信仰。（take into consideration/account）

_____

4. 无论你是在服用处方药还是非处方药，重要的是按照说明用药，并且只用于药物的预期用途。（whether）

_____

5. 保持有效期还能帮助你避免服用无效药物。（keep up with）

_____

Listening & Speaking

Task 1　David is an overseas student in China. Today, he is talking about Chinese medicine with his classmate Liu Yang, who is a native Chinese. Listen to the conversation and decide whether the following statements are true（T）or false（F）.

Overseas Students in China：Chinese Medicine

（　）1. David and Liu Yang are overseas students in China.

（　）2. Chinese people are more accustomed to Chinese medicine.

（　）3. Chinese medicine strives to bring balance to the body as a whole.

（　）4. Chinese medicine only accounts for 20% ~ 25% of the whole pharmaceutical market.

（　）5. David prefers western medicine.

📖 **Notes**

1. Are Chinese people more accustomed to Chinese medicine?

中国人更习惯服用中药吗？

Listening & Speaking Task 1

be accustomed to　习惯于；适应于。

e. g. More and more people will be accustomed to it.

越来越多的人会习惯于它。

2. in contrast/by comparison　与此相反；相比之下。

e. g. In contrast, education can actually transform a nation.

相反，实际上教育能转变一个国家。

3. wholesome adj. 适合；卫生的；有益健康的；显示身心健康的。

e. g. It is not wholesome to eat without washing your hands.

不洗手吃饭是不卫生的。

4. the whole pharmaceutical market　整个医药市场。

Task 2　**As a pharmacist, you are not only familiar with the classification of drugs, but also responsible for the reviewing and supervision of prescription dispensing. Listen to the conversation and choose the best answer to each question you hear.**

I Need to Refill This Prescription

(　) 1. How many times can this prescription be refilled up?

　　A. Once　　　　　　　　B. Twice

　　C. Three times　　　　　D. None

(　) 2. What was this prescription for?

　　A. Mental　　　　　　　B. Skin

　　C. Heart　　　　　　　D. Skeletal muscle

(　) 3. Why didn't the patient's doctor write her a new prescription?

　　A. Because he was unhappy　　B. Because she got a new doctor

　　C. Becausehe was out of town　D. We didn't know

(　) 4. Why didn't the pharmacist refill the patient's prescription?

　　A. Because he didn't like her

　　B. Because there were other pharmacists

　　C. Because it is illegal to sell drugs without a prescription

　　D. All are true

(　) 5. According to the conversation, which statement is not correct?

　　A. The patient's prescription has already been refilled twice

　　B. The patient has run out of this prescription

　　C. The patient's prescription has expired

　　D. The pharmacist refilled up the patient's prescription

📖 **Notes**

1. against the law　违法的，犯法的。

e. g. Concealment of evidence is against the law.

隐藏证据是违法的。

2. A prescription must be valid. It cannot be an expired prescription.

处方必须是有效的，不可以是过期的处方。

3. I have a special medical plan.

我有特殊的医疗方案。

4. frustrating adj. 令人沮丧的。

e. g. The current situation is very frustrating for us.

目前的局势对我们来讲是很令人懊丧的。

Task 3   **It is very useful for us pharmaceutical students to understand the nature of work in pharmacy. Listen to the following passage and fill in the blanks with what you hear.**

Listening &
Speaking
Task 3

Pharmacy-Health-Prescription

I recently graduated from a pharmacy school. Now I work as a staff pharmacist in a local drug store. My __1__ has a Doctor of Pharmacy degree. He __2__ the entire operation. Although it is a rather small pharmacy, we do carry most of the prescription drugs on a daily basis. In case the __3__ drugs are not available in stock; I can usually place an order for them in less than 24 hours. Most of our clients are senior citizens. Some of them come in quite frequently, and the most prescribed drug is the __4__. I have learned how to file prescription insurance claims, divide drugs into small packages, and locate the right direction labels for the pills. I take my job very __5__ because it directly affects people's health. A responsible attitude is a must because any careless mistakes can lead to grave consequences.

Task 4   **Work in groups, try to discuss the differences and connections between Rx and OTC, Chinese and western medicine. Practice making the conversations with your partner according to what you hear in the Listening part.**

Partner A	Partner B
Greet as usual.	Ask about the sale of prescription drugs.
Explain the rule.	Then talk about the differences between Rx and OTC.
Also supplement the connections.	Express the interest in Chinese medicine.
Compare Chinese medicine with Western medicine.	Show respect for medicine, and to study pharmacy well.
Agree with the point.	Say goodbye.

Reading B

Classification of Drugs

Introduction to Drugs

Drugs, the word is not new to us. However, the word generally creates a frightful response amongst many. So far, we have heard that drugs are the substance of addiction and a reason for the spoiled generation. This is mainly because people have been abusing the substance which has led to the death of even popular people as well.

Yes, they are addictive but did you know that all of them are not harmful. Biologically speaking, drugs mostly target our brains and switch the mood and physiological conditions of our bodies. However, since there are various types of drugs including legal as well as illegal drugs, the latter is causing most of the problems.

Having said that, on this page we will be discussing mainly the legal drugs and their classifications.

What Are Drugs?

By definition, drugs are chemical substances that affect or alter the physiology when taken into a living system. They can either be natural or synthetic.

Chemically, they are low atomic mass and molecular mass structures. When a drug is therapeutically active and is used for the diagnosis, treatment or prevention of a disease, it is called medicine (legal drugs). They target the macromolecules inside the body and generate a biological response. Most of them interrupt the nervous system (especially brain) for the generation of a proper biological response. However, they can be toxic in higher doses and generally referred to as lethal dose.

Classification of Drugs

Classification of drugs can be done on the basis of certain criteria. Some of them are given below.

· Classification of Drugs on the Basis of the Pharmacological Effect

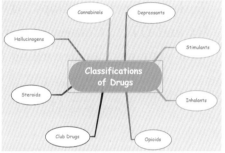

How a drug or medicine affects or influences the cells of an organism is referred to as the pharmacological effect. Different types of drugs have various pharmacological effects on an organism. For example, an analgesic reduces pain while an anti-inflammatory drug reduces the inflammation of the body. Thus, drugs can be classified based on the pharmacological effect.

· Classification of Drugs on the Basis of Drug Action

Different drugs act differently, i. e. each drug has its own way of generating a response called drug action. Drug action is more specified according to how it generates a response. For example, there are lots of medicines to treat hypertension, but each type of drug has different drug actions. All the hypertension medicines reduce the blood pressure but in a different pathway.

· Classification of Drugs on the Basis of Chemical Structure

This is a common classification of drugs. Generally, drugs that have the same drug action and pharmacological effect have a basic skeletal structure and a minute variation in the branching. This is why some drugs have more potential than the others. For example, all sulphonamides have the same skeletal structure.

· Classification of Drugs on the Basis of Molecular Targets

Drugs target the macromolecules inside the body to generate a biological response. Such macromolecules are called target molecules or drug targets. Drugs that have the same mechanism of action will have the same target. This basis for the classification of drugs is more helpful during clinical trials.

(517 words)

Words and Expressions

classification	/ˌklæsifiˈkeiʃn/	n.	分类；类别，等级
frightful	/ˈfraitfl/	adj.	可怕的；惊人的；非常的
amongst	/əˈmʌŋst/	prep.	在……当中（= among）
addiction	/əˈdikʃn/	n.	上瘾，沉溺；癖嗜
spoiled	/spɔild/	adj.	（尤指小孩）被宠坏的
abuse	/əˈbjuːs/	vt.	滥用；虐待；辱骂
		n.	滥用；虐待；辱骂；弊端
addictive	/əˈdiktiv/	adj.	使人上瘾的
target	/ˈtɑːgit/	v.	把……作为目标；面向
		n.	（攻击的）对象；靶子
synthetic	/sinˈθetik/	adj.	综合的；合成的，人造的
		n.	合成物
atomic	/əˈtɒmik/	adj.	原子的；微粒子的
mass	/mæs/	n.	块；民众；大量；质量
		adj.	群众的；集中的
molecular	/məˈlekjələ(r)/	adj.	分子的；由分子组成的
therapeutically	/ˌθerəˈpjuːtikli/	adv.	在治疗上；有疗效地
macromolecule	/ˌmækrə(ʊ)ˈmɒlikjuːl/	n.	高分子；[化学]大分子
generate	/ˈdʒenəreit/	vt.	生殖；产生物理反应
toxic	/ˈtɒksik/	adj.	有毒的；中毒的
lethal	/ˈliːθl/	adj.	致命的，致死的
pharmacological	/ˌfɑːməkəˈlɒdʒikl/	adj.	药理学的
analgesic	/ˌænəlˈdʒiːzik/	n.	镇痛剂
anti-inflammatory	/ˌæntiinˈflæmətri/	adj.	抗炎的
hypertension	/ˌhaipəˈtenʃn/	n.	高血压；过度紧张
pathway	/ˈpɑːθwei/	n.	道；路径；神经通路
skeletal	/ˈskelətl/	adj.	骨骼的；骨瘦如柴的
branching	/ˈbræntʃiŋ/	n.	分支；分歧
sulphonamides	/sʌlfəˈnæmaid/	n.	磺胺；磺胺类药剂
molecule	/ˈmɒlikjuːl/	n.	[化学]分子；微粒
trials	/ˈtraiəl/	n.	试验；审讯；努力；磨炼
living system		生命系统	
lethal dose		致死剂量	
pharmacological effect		药理效应	
molecular targets		分子靶点	

Proper Names

physiological conditions	[生理]生理条件
i. e.	也就是，亦即（源自拉丁文 id est）

After-reading Exercises

Task 1 Read the passage and choose the correct answer to each question.

(   ) 1. According to the passagehow many classifications of drugs can be done?

    A. Two   B. Three

    C. Four   D. Five

(   ) 2. Which of the following are the biological effects of drugs?

    A. Our brains   B. Our emotions

    C. Our physiology   D. All of the above

(   ) 3. Which drug can reduce the inflammation of the body?

    A. An analgesic   B. An anti-inflammatory drug

    C. All the hypertension medicines   D. All sulphonamides

(   ) 4. Which of the following statements is not true?

    A. All of drug is harmful

    B. Drugs are addictive

    C. There are natural and synthetic drugs

    D. There are legal and illegal drugs

(   ) 5. Which classification of drugs is more helpful during clinical trials?

    Classification of Drugs on the basis of the _____ .

    A. pharmacological Effect   B. drug Action

    C. chemical Structure   D. molecular Targets

Task 2 Translate the following sentences into Chinese.

1. Biologically speaking, drugs mostly target our brains and switch the mood and physiological conditions of our bodies.

_____

2. By definition, drugs are chemical substances that affect or alter the physiology when taken into a living system.

_____

3. For example, an analgesic reduces pain while an anti-inflammatory drug reduces the inflammation of the body.

_____

4. Different drugs act differently, i. e. each drug has its own way of generating a response called drug action.

_____

5. This basis for the classification of drugs is more helpful during clinical trials.

_____

Practical Writing

Resume

求职简历又称求职资历、个人履历等，是求职者将自己与所申请职位紧密相关的个人信息经过分析整理并清晰简要地表述出来的书面求职资料，是一种应用写作文体。在这里求职者用真实准确的事实向招聘者明示自己的经历、经验、技能、成果等内容。求职简历是招聘者在阅读求职者求职申请后对其产生兴趣，进而进一步决定是否给予面试机会的极重要的依据性材料。

英文简历写作技巧

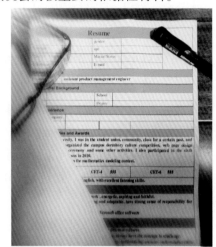

1. Personal Information（个人信息）：姓名、地址、联系方式、电话、电子邮箱等。

2. Objective（求职意向）：这一栏是最重要的一项了。很多公司主要看这一项的内容是否跟他们所要求的一致或者接近。

3. Summary（个人简介）：展现个人能力的好机会，既要赞美自己，又不能让对方觉得你在自夸。

4. Work/Career Experience（工作经验）：如果工作经验很多，没有必要完全列举出来，可以挑几项自己感觉最满意的或者对自己提升最大的来写。按照时间由近及远的顺序写。

5. Educational Background（教育背景）：一般从大学开始写起，包括时间、学校、专业、学位、奖项，尤其是特殊奖项等。

6. 自选内容。比如：Associations（社团组织）、Computer background（计算机能力）、Language Skills（外语水平）、Marital Status（婚姻情况）、Health（身体状况）、Hobbies（业余爱好）、Personal Profile（个人评价）等。

Sample

Resume

Name：Chen Yan　Sex：Female　Age：37

Address：Suite 1, No. 2, Lane, East Haiyang Road, Shanghai

Mobile：13800138000　E-mail：chenyan@ sina. com

Educational Background：

2006-2008：had studied at pharmaceutical research institute of Gauvin University, Japan, and obtained a master's degree.

2001-2005：had studied specialty of bio-chemistry at East China Science University, and obtained a bachelor's degree.

Career Experience：

2015-now：has acted as a senior manager of medicine manufacturing division of a big-sized group enterprise the "China Chaoyang Group Corp."

2014-2015：had acted as the general manager of Shanghai Technology Co. Ltd.（an individual-owned company）, in charge of overall management affairs of selling the imported medicinal additives on the home market.

2010-2013：had been a Chinese marketing manager of medicine and food additives division of a famous big-sized Japanese company.

2008-2009：had been a visiting scholar at Pha Zd.

Task　You are required to fill in the Resume according to the following information given in Chinese. Then work in groups to discuss the requirements and precautions about English resumes for us as fresh graduates in the future and make a complete Resume in English for yourself.

刘洋，男，生于 1992 年 5 月 12 日。家住南方市东海路 65 号，联系电话为 15312345678，电子邮箱 liuyang@ qq. com。申请药品销售主管一职。

从 2006 年 9 月至 2009 年 7 月就读南方市第一中学。自 2009 年 9 月至 2012 年 7 月在江南职业技术学院学习，药学专业。曾获得 2010、2011 年度奖学金，并于 2011 年通过计算机考试，获得证书。

大学毕业后就职于 ABC 公司，负责药品销售与管理。熟悉办公室工作，能熟练使用电脑。工作期间，接受过国内与国外的技术培训。

善于沟通，能很好地与团队成员合作。热爱足球和摄影。

Resume

Name：Liu Yang　Sex：＿＿＿＿＿＿　Date of Birth：＿＿＿＿＿＿

Address：No. 65, Donghai Road, Nanfang

Mobile：15312345678　E-mail：liuyang@ qq. com

Position Applied for：＿＿＿＿＿＿

Educational Background：

Sept. 2009-July 2012：＿＿＿＿＿＿＿＿＿＿ .

＿＿＿＿＿＿＿＿＿＿ .

＿＿＿＿＿＿＿＿＿＿ .

Sept. 2006-July 2009：Studied in No. 1 High School of Nanfang.

Work Experience：

July 2012-now：＿＿＿＿＿＿＿＿＿＿ .

＿＿＿＿＿＿＿＿＿＿ .

＿＿＿＿＿＿＿＿＿＿ .

Strong Points：＿＿＿＿＿＿＿＿＿＿ .

Hobbies：Football and Photographing

Grammar Tips

简单句就是只含有一个主谓结构，并且句子各成分都只由单词或短语构成的独立句子或分句。在简单句中主语和谓语是句子的主干，是句子的核心。

Simple Sentences

根据句子结构分类：五大基本句型

句型	例句
主语 + 不及物动词（S + Vi）	We all breathe, eat, and drink.
主语 + 及物动词 + 宾语（S + Vt + DO）	We should study Medicine.
主语 + 系动词 + 表语（S + Link-V + P）	This is an English-Chinese dictionary.
主语 + 及物动词 + 间接宾语 + 直接宾语（S + Vt + IO + DO）	The doctor gave me some pills.
主语 + 及物动词 + 宾语 + 宾语补足语（S + Vt + O + OC）	We will keep the patient awake.

根据句子作用分类：四大句型

句型		例句
陈述句	肯定句	They like skating.
	否定句	He didn't go shopping yesterday.
疑问句	一般疑问句	Are you interested in TCM?
	特殊疑问句	How many books are there in the room?
	选择疑问句	Does your son work in the drug shop or a company?
	反意疑问句	You can't swim, can you?
祈使句	肯定祈使句	Practice speaking English every day.
	否定祈使句	Don't be afraid of making mistakes.
感叹句	What 引导	What hardworking students I am teaching!
	How 引导	How hot and wet the weather is today!

Task 1   Mark the types of the following simple sentences with a formula.

1. Anna speaks Russian. _____

2. Daddy bought Tom a new dictionary. _____

3. Kate calls her cat Mimi. _____

4. Polly laughed. _____

5. Lily felt cold. _____

6. The picture looks beautiful. _____

7. Jim brought me my English books. _____

8. It is dangerous. _____

9. You must wait. _____

10. Mr. Green can't keep the house tidy. _____

Task 2 Choose the best answer to complete each sentence according to Simple Sentences.

(   ) 1. The sign here says "No parking". Why _____ your car in the underground parking lot?

       A. not park   B. don't park

       C. not parking   D. aren't parking

(   ) 2. ——Hey, Shirley, welcome back! _____?

       ——Ok, I guess. My son and I went to Hainan and enjoyed the beautiful scenery there.

       A. How was your holiday

       B. How is your son

       C. Where did you go for holiday

       D. What did you do in your holiday

(   ) 3. _____ it is to skate on real ice!

       A. What fun   B. What a fun

       C. How a fun   D. What funs

(   ) 4. Taking exercise every morning helps to lose weight, _____?

       A. doesn't it   B. don't they

       C. isn't it   D. aren't they

(   ) 5. On Sunday I often stay at home and do some _____ .

       A. read   B. reads

       C. reading   D. to read

(   ) 6. You must have seen him off yesterday, _____?

       A. haven't you   B. didn't you

       C. mustn't you   D. needn't you

(   ) 7. _____ useful information it is!

       A. How   B. What

       C. What a   D. How a

(   ) 8. ——English has a large vocabulary, hasn't it?

       ——Yes. _____ more words and expressions and you will find it easier to read and communicate.

       A. Know   B. Knowing

       C. To know   D. Having known

(   ) 9. _____ role she played in the movie! No wonder she has won an Oscar.

       A. How interesting   B. How an interesting

       C. What interesting   D. What an interesting

(   ) 10. The teacher told her students _____ in public.

       A. not to shout   B. didn't shout

       C. not shout   D. to not shout

Supplementary Reading

Understanding Chinese Medicine and Western Medicine to Reach the Maximum Treatment Benefit

Chuanhai Cao and Brown B.

Medicine can be traced back to as early as the origin of man, since food and medicine are intertwined. Some foods can be used for medicinal purposes, and some foods with medicinal properties are also used as everyday foods. This is very much true of herbal medicine.

When we moved towards industrialization, modern Western medicine became the dominant medical practices. Since then, herbal medicine gradually lost its dominant position in disease treatment. We are challenged by the choice of using traditional medicine or modern medicine. Traditional medicine, known as Traditional Chinese Medicine, includes surgery, moxibustion, hot cupping, acupuncture, massage, herbal medicine and nutraceutical medicine. Modern medicine, known as Western medicine, includes surgery and most commonly single molecular drugs.

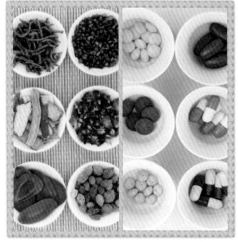

The Major Differences between Western Medicine and Chinese Medicine

Chinese medicine diagnoses through the symptoms of the patient described and appearances (eye, skin and tongue color as well as pulse), then seeks to address the overall systemic problem with a focus on preventing any potential adverse effects.

Western medicine treats symptoms and treats the target or target organ as isolated from the rest of the body instead of as one whole interconnected system.

Western medicine provides diagnosis through lab test and it focuses on eliminating symptoms but normally fails to address adverse effects on the body.

Chinese medicine focuses on the body's overall response to treatment and recognizes the body as one interconnected biosystem. Treatment changes the overall condition of the body including the immune system, but also takes care of the specific target problem.

Onset Time of Drugs

Western medicine typically has rapid or immediate effects, so it is highly effective for life-threatening conditions. However, the major issue associated with these drugs is the potential damage they may have to other parts of body even though it is a life-saving procedure or method.

Chinese medicine is designed to both prevent adverse effects and treat diseases. The onset of drug efficacy compared to Western medicine is longer, but it is safer to use, since it takes into account potential adverse effects. It can also prevent the secondary or aftereffects caused by treatments seen in Western medicine.

Maximum Treatment Benefits Combining Western and Chinese Medicine

There is a principle of traditional medicine called "Jun-Chen-Zuo-Shi" which covers four functions:

1. Denominator or Key Element：A drug or a molecule that directly fights or targets the pathological factor related to a disease.

2. Assistant or Enhancer：A drug or a molecule that can enhance the function of the drug.

3. Corrector or Addresser of Adverse Effects：A drug or a molecule that can prevent adverse effects that are related to the denominator or enhancer in order to limit abnormal responses.

4. Messenger：A drug or a molecule that can bring the function of the denominator to the target site.

It is not inherently good or bad to use one method or the other to treat disease. We believe the best treatment approach to use to treat human disease should follow the principle of Chinese medicine "Jun-Chen-Zhou-Shi". It is a combination therapy using Western medicine to alleviate current symptoms and using Chinese medicine concurrently to address the root cause of the disease as well as preventing disease reoccurrence. This method uses Western medicine as a key element, and the Chinese medicinal approach serves as an assistant addresser and messenger.

(Department of Pharmaceutical Sciences, College of Pharmacy, University of South Florida, MDC4106A 12901 Bruce B. Downs Blvd, Tampa FL 33612, USA)

(591 words)

After-reading Exercises

Task Decide whether the following statements are true (T) or false (F) according to the text.

(   ) 1. Herbal medicine has no position in disease treatment.

(   ) 2. Western medicine diagnoses through eye, skin and tongue color as well as pulse.

(   ) 3. There is a principle of traditional medicine called "Jun-Chen-Zuo-Shi".

(   ) 4. Chinese medicine is highly effective for life-threatening conditions.

(   ) 5. It is not inherently good or bad to use one method or the other to treat disease.

Vocabulary Tips

Root "optic-"：眼的。来自拉丁语 opticus, 眼睛的，来自希腊语 ops, 眼睛。

Example：optical adj. 眼的；optician 眼睛和光学仪器制造者；optics 光学；optometer 视力计 optometrist 验光师；optometry 视力测定。

Root "all-, allo-"：另外的，异。来源于拉丁语 alius。

Example：allergy 过敏症，反感，厌恶；allergic 过敏的；allergen 过敏原；allogamy 异花受粉（受精）；allopathy 对抗疗法；allograph 别人代笔的文件。

Prefix "hyper-"：超过的，高。来源于希腊语 hyper 和拉丁语 hyper-。

Example：hypertension 过度紧张，高血压（hyper + tension 紧张）；hypersensitive 过敏的（hyper + sensitive 敏感的）；hyperacid 胃酸过多的。

Task Complete the sentences with the given words.

allergen	hypersensitive	optical	optics	allopathic

1. _____ technology is one of the most sensational developments in recent years.

2. Your body may have a threshold（界限）for a particular _____, such as pollen or animal dander（动物的皮屑）.

3. These _____ fibres may be used for new sorts of telephony.

4. We have tried various medications（_____ and homeopathic 对抗疗法，顺势疗法）, but they have not helped.

5. The skin on various parts of the body becomes _____.

Proverbs and Sayings

◇Prescribe the right medicine for a symptom.

对症下药。

◇Get busy. Keep busy. It's the cheapest kind of medicine there is on this earth — and one of the best.

忙起来吧，一直忙碌着，这是世界上最便宜也是最有效的药物。

◇One of the first duties of the physician is to educate the masses not to take medicine.

医生的首要职责之一是教育人们不要吃药。

题库

Unit 4

Chinese Materia Medica

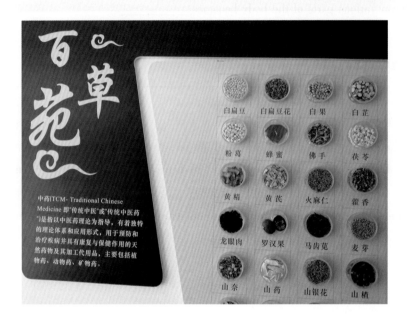

Unit Objectives

After studying this unit, you are expected to:

· master the vocabulary and technical terms related to Chinese materia medica;

· understand the history of Chinese materia medica and its future;

· know noun clauses correctly.

And you should learn how to:

· communicate with others about the decocting methods and Cordyceps;

· write a company profile.

Introduction

Chinese materia medica has been used as a major tool in traditional Chinese medicine to treat disorders. Generally, it includes oral administration (usually prepared into decoction, pill, powder, decocted extract, and medicinal wine) and external application (including moxa-compression, medicinal bath, laryngeal insufflation, eye dropping, warm medicated compression, and suppository).

In ancient Chinese materia medica works, there are many records about prohibited combination like mutual antagonism and mutual incompatibility, which should be used with more cautions.

Warming-up

Task　Work in groups. Match the pictures to the proper statements.
Then check your answers with your partner.

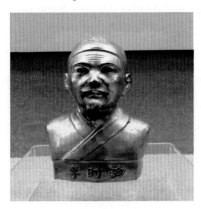

A

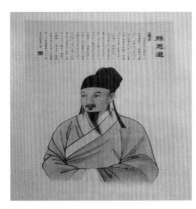

B

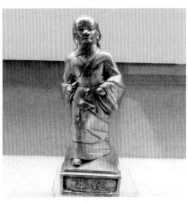

C

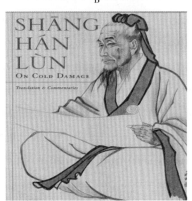

D

(　) 1. He was titled as China's King of Medicine for his significant contributions to Chinese medicine and tremendous care to his patients.

(　) 2. His major contribution to clinical medicine was his 27-year work, which is found in his scientific book *Compendium of Materia Medica*.

(　) 3. He was a Chinese physician who wrote in the early 3rd century a work titled *Shang han za bing lun* (*Treatise on Febrile and Other Diseases*).

(　) 4. He was the first person in China to use anaesthesia during surgery, which is called *Mafeisan*. In addition, he developed the *Wuqinxi* from studying movements of the tiger, deer, bear, ape and crane.

医药大学堂
WWW.YIYAODXT.COM

Reading A

Chinese Materia Medica and Its Science

Chinese materia medica refers to the botanical, mineral, and zoological substances applied by traditional Chinese medicine as a primary weapon for preventing and treating diseases. Some people are of the wrong impression that Chinese materia medica are all produced in China. However, some medical substances are either from other parts of the world or have been introduced and planted in China.

Back in early history when people relied on collecting plants and hunting animals as their main source of food, they gradually recognized the beneficial or harmful effects of those plants or animals on human body. This is the original knowledge of Chinese materia medica. With a time-honored history of civilization tracing back to 6000 years ago, China has a large population, vast territory, and abundant resources. Chinese people have accumulated rich medical experience in fighting for survival and disease prevention and treatment, and gradually built up the theoretical knowledge of Chinese materia medica. About 2000 years ago when *The Yellow Emperor's Inner Classic* and *Shen Nong's Classic of the Materia Medica* have been compiled, a comprehensive theoretical system of Chinese materia medica has formed. The former is a systematical expression of the correlative theories of Chinese materia medica and principles of their application, such as four natures, five flavors, relations between the five-zang organs and medical natures and flavors, and medicinal selection for five-zang organs' diseases, while the latter focuses on the detailed description of 365 herbs in terms of natures, flavors, actions, and indications.

Science of Chinese materia medica, as one of the primary disciplines of traditional Chinese medicine, mainly expounds the basic knowledge of Chinese medicine in terms of source, nature, processing, actions, indications, as well as its basic theories and administration.

In ancient China, Science of Chinese materia medica and correlative works were called "materia medica" because herbal medicine is a major component. There are abundant books on materia medica in history with a continuous accretion of new herbs together with a revaluation and addition of new uses, which is a reflection of China's wealth. China is rich in Chinese medicinal resources and science of Chinese materia medica is rich in content with great numbers of Chinese medicinals.

With great achievements, Science of Chinese materia medica not only plays an essential role in the historical development of traditional Chinese medicine in China and medicine in neighboring countries, but also has exerted important influences on the development of medicine across the world. Studies on Chinese materia medica, especially crude medicinals, become one of the hotspots in the international medical fields and new products are

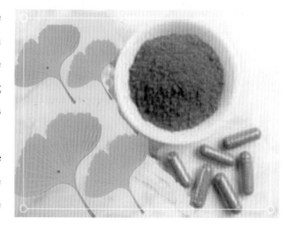

extracted from Chinese medicinals every year. For instance, medicines prepared from active ingredients extracted from Yín Xìng Yè (Folium Ginkgo, ginkgo leaf), which is known for its excellent actions of preventing and treating cardiovascular diseases, bring great profits to European pharmaceutical companies.

(527 words)

Words and Expressions

weapon	/ˈwepən/	n.	手段
beneficial	/beniˈfiʃl/	adj.	有益的
territory	/ˈterətri/	n.	领土
abundant	/əˈbʌndənt/	adj.	丰富的
accumulate	/əˈkjuːmjəleit/	vt.	积累
medical	/ˈmedikl/	adj.	医学的；药的；内科的
survival	/səˈvaivl/	n.	（在困境中的）生存
theoretical	/ˌθiəˈretikl/	adj.	理论的；理论上的
systematical	/ˌsistəˈmætikl/	adj.	系统的
correlative	/kəˈrelətiv/	adj.	相关的
nature	/ˈneitʃə(r)/	n.	性质；本性
action	/ˈækʃn/	n.	作用；功能
indication	/ˌindiˈkeiʃn/	n.	适应证
discipline	/ˈdisəplin/	n.	学科
expound	/ikˈspaʊnd/	v.	阐述；讲解
processing	/prəʊsesiŋ/	n.	加工
administration	/ədˌminiˈstreiʃn/	n.	管理；实施
component	/kəmˈpəʊnənt/	n.	组成部分
accretion	/əˈkriːʃn/	n.	积聚；积淀物
revaluation	/ˌriːvæljuˈeiʃn/	n.	重新估价；再评价
reflection	/riˈflekʃn/	n.	反映
medicinal	/məˈdisinl/	adj.	药的；药用的；治疗的
essential	/iˈsenʃl/	adj.	基本的；必要的；本质的
exert	/igˈzɜːt/	v.	运用，发挥；施以影响
crude	/kruːd/	adj.	天然的，未加工的
hotspot	/hɒtspɒt/	n.	热点
extract	/ˈekstrækt/	vt.	提取，提炼
cardiovascular	/ˌkɑːdiəʊˈvæskjələ(r)/	adj.	心血管的

Proper Names

Chinese materia medica	中药
Folium Ginkgo	银杏叶，即 ginkgo leaf

📖 Notes

1. Chinese materia medica refers to the botanical, mineral, and zoological substances applied by traditional Chinese medicine as a primary weapon for preventing and treating diseases.

中药包括植物药、动物药和矿物药，是中医预防、治疗疾病的主要手段。

applied by⋯是过去分词短语做后置定语，修饰 substances。

2. Some people are of the wrong impression that Chinese materia medica are all produced in China.

一些人误认为中药都产自中国。

"that"引导同位语从句，修饰 the wrong impression。

3. With a time-honored history of civilization tracing back to 6000 years ago…

悠久的文明史可以追溯到 6000 年前。

time-honored，历史悠久的，tracing back…，追溯到……相当于 dating back to，

这里是现在分词短语做后置定语，相当于定语从句"which traces back…"。

4. The former is a systematical…, while the latter focuses on the detailed description of 365 herbs in terms of natures, flavors, actions, and indications.

前者（《黄帝内经》）系统表述了中药学相关理论及其应用原则，如"四气五味"、五脏与"气、味的关系"、五脏疾病的药物选择等；后者（《神农本草经》）则详细描述了 365 种草药的"性味"、作用及适应证。

"while"，连词，翻译成"然而"，还有"当…时"的含义，亦可作名词，有词组 after a while，翻译成"过了一会儿"。

e. g. Their country has plenty of oil, while ours has none.

他们的国家盛产石油，而我们国家却一点也没有。

5. Science of Chinese Materia Medica, as one of the primary disciplines of traditional Chinese medicine, … as well as its basic theories and administration.

作为中医药的基础学科，中药学主要介绍了中药的基础理论和施用，还介绍了中药的来源、性状、炮制、作用、适应证等方面的基础知识。

"as well as…"，意为"除……之外；也；还"，相当于 in addition to sb/sth; too。

e. g. They sell books as well as newspapers.

他们既卖报也卖书。

6. … medicines prepared from active ingredients extracted from Yín Xìng Yè（Folium Ginkgo, ginkgo leaf），which is known for its excellent actions of preventing and treating cardiovascular diseases,

……银杏叶提取物以其预防和治疗心血管疾病的功效而闻名，欧洲制药企业因此获得了巨额利润。

"prepared from active ingredients"，过去分词做后置定语修饰 medicines，"which is known for…"，非限制性定语从句，修饰 Yín Xìng Yè。

After-reading Exercises

Task 1　Answer the following questions according to the text.

1. What is Chinese materia medica?

_____

2. Are Chinese materia medica all produced in China?

_____

3. When did the system of Chinese materia medica begin to form?

_____

4. What are the main contents of science of Chinese materia medica?

_____

5. What is the action of ginkgo leaf?

_____

Task 2   Match the words（1-10）to the Chinese meanings（a-j）.

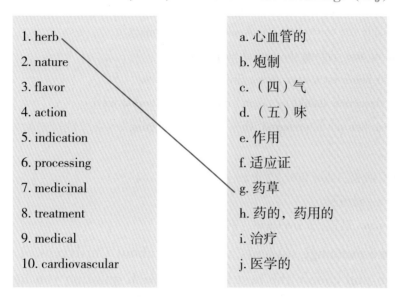

1. herb   a. 心血管的

2. nature   b. 炮制

3. flavor   c.（四）气

4. action   d.（五）味

5. indication   e. 作用

6. processing   f. 适应证

7. medicinal   g. 药草

8. treatment   h. 药的，药用的

9. medical   i. 治疗

10. cardiovascular j. 医学的

Task 3   Fill in each blank with the proper form of the word or phrase given in brackets.

1. He is receiving _____ for shock.（treat）

2. Heavy bleeding is a common _____ for hysterectomy（子宫切除术）.（indicate）

3. He keeps a bottle of brandy only for _____ purposes.（medicine）

4. She is the lady who chose _____ childbirth.（nature）

5. This is a study of the _____ of the liver.（act）

Task 4   Translate the following sentences into English using the words or phrases you have learned in this unit.

1. 一些人误认为中药都产自中国。（be of the wrong impression that…）

_____

2. 中药已成为中医治疗疾病的主要工具。（Chinese materia medica）

_____

3. 中国人民积累了丰富的医学经验。（medical experience）

_____

4. 中药学在中医药发展史上起着重要作用。（play an essential role in）

_____

5. 银杏叶以其防治心血管疾病的功效而闻名。（be known for）

_____

Listening & Speaking

Listening &
Speaking
Task 1

Task 1 A pharmacist is filling the prescription for a patient. Listen to the conversation and decide whether the following statements are true(T) or false(F).

Could You Fill the Prescription for Me?

(   ) 1. Probably the conversation took place in a pharmacy.

(   ) 2. It is no use soaking the herbal medicine.

(   ) 3. You'd better cook over strong fire for 13 minutes.

(   ) 4. The decoction should be taken, including the herbal leaves.

(   ) 5. An earthen pot is preferred when you are decocting.

📖 **Notes**

1. strong fire　武火；slow fire　文火。

2. decoction　一剂汤药。

3. an earthen pot　砂锅；a steel pan　钢锅。

Listening &
Speaking
Task 2

Task 2 Two exchange students are talking about Cordyceps. Listen to the conversation and choose the best answer to each question you hear.

Cordyceps

(   ) 1. What does Cordyceps look like?

　　A. Interesting　　　　　　　　B. Normal

　　C. Queer　　　　　　　　　　D. Not mentioned

(   ) 2. Where can Cordyceps grow?

　　A. In England　　　　　　　　B. Only in China

　　C. In Europe　　　　　　　　D. In Asia

(   ) 3. The action of Cordyceps is to cure ailments, such as _____.

　　A. night sweat　　　　　　　　B. pain at waist and knees

　　C. anaemia　　　　　　　　　D. All of the above.

(   ) 4. Does Cordyceps have side effect?

　　A. No

　　B. Not mentioned

　　C. Yes. Cordyceps has a lot of side effects

　　D. It is unknown whether Cordyceps has side effects or not

(   ) 5. Is there anything you mustn't eat when taking Cordyceps?

　　A. Duck　　　　　　　　　　B. Chicken

　　C. Garlic　　　　　　　　　　D. Nothing

📖 **Notes**

1. Cordyceps　冬虫夏草，也称作 cordyceps sinensis。

2. besides　而且，另外，同义词组：in addition, what's more, one more thing。

医药大学堂
WWW.YIYAODXT.COM

Listening &
Speaking
Task 3

Task 3 **The use of Chinese medicinals is common in our life. Listen to the following passage and fill in the blanks with what you hear.**

Jinhua Qinggan Granule was developed during the 2009 H1N1 influenza _____1_____. It consists of 12 herbal components including honeysuckle, mint and licorice and can _____2_____ heat and detoxify lungs. It has a curative effect in treating _____3_____ and moderate patients and can also improve the _____4_____ of lymphocyte and white blood cells as well as reduce the rate of patients turning more severe. A comparative experiment showed that patients who took Jinhua Qinggan Granule tested _____5_____ for coronavirus two and a half days earlier than a group that did not take the granule. The group treated with the granule also took eight days to show improvement, while the other group took 10.3 days.

Task 4 **Work in groups, try to discuss the topic of "Could you fill the prescription for me?" and "Cordyceps". Practice making the conversations with your partner according to what you hear in the Listening part.**

Partner A (pharmacist)	Partner B (patient)
Greet.	Greet and ask for the prescription.
Make up the prescription.	Ask how to decoct Chinese herbs.
Explain the way of decocting.	Talk about the dos and don'ts.
Give further explanation.	Confirm information.
Express a wish for recovery.	Show the appreciation.

Reading B

Chinese Medicine: the Battle for Acceptance

The global medical community has debated the efficacy of traditional Chinese medicine for decades. In the midst of the still-unfolding novel coronavirus pandemic, traditional Chinese medicine (TCM) has once again become the bone of contention. While a set of Chinese patent drugs have proven effective in treating mildly symptomatic patients, Western medical communities are skeptical, citing a dearth of rigorous trial data to question their clinical efficacy.

Faced with this new, elusive virus that caught the world off guard, major countries are all working on the scientific frontier to develop clinical protocols in the absence of a widely recognized vaccine. Chinese medicine makes up 111 out of all the 345 protocols put forward by China. Just like in the past, the "historical experience" has again gone under scrutiny.

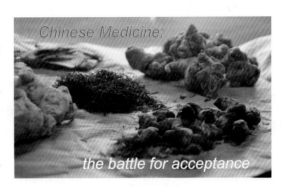

Chinese Medicine: the battle for acceptance

The first attempt to put Chinese medicine on the global market dates back to 1997 when makers of a drug used to treat coronary heart disease, called "Compound Danshen Dripping Pill", was submitted for approval by the U. S. Food and Drug Administration (FDA). Since then, more than 10 Chinese patent drugs have made attempts, but only three have made it into Phase III clinical trials——Compound Danshen Dripping Pills, HMPL-004 and Xuezhikang.

The FDA issued a draft Botanical Drug Development Guidance for Industry in 2004 and finalized it in 2016. The guide says since botanical drugs may remain as complex mixtures, "Both purification and identification of the active ingredients in botanicals are optional and not required." It also states that clinical information from the extensive human use of botanical products can be used in new drug development and regulatory review.

Western medicine is based on the science of pharmacology and toxicology while TCM is more empirically-based through a history of thousands of years. Chinese herbal medicines have complex chemical makeups, and thus require a lot of effort to understand which component is effective, and how components interact with each other to contribute to alleviating certain symptoms.

To enhance the global presence of Chinese medicine, the most important factors are strong science, consensus, quality, and investment in relevant clinical studies. Understanding the benefits of Chinese medicine and leveraging its use in conjunction with Western remedies are key to increasing global acceptance for herbal drugs. With the whole COVID-19 epidemic, there's a very good combination of Chinese and Western medicines being used. But building science behind drug products is very important, and we are generating more data for efficacy.

The coronavirus disease has stoked Western countries' interest in TCM, but it remains hard for TCM to gain traction worldwide. People are not that optimistic about widespread recognition of Chinese medicine. But at least, they have come to know that Chinese medicine can treat acute viral infections through the pandemic. China's come a long way in regulating TCM plantation and marketing, and now relevant products have reached a qualification rate of over 80 percent. More needs to be done.

The role of Chinese medicine will increase. Chinese medicine has its uniqueness and advantages, especially in preventing and treating chronic diseases. It has a strong fit when we look at the macro trend of an aging population.

The internationalization of TCM will happen, it is just a matter of when.

(572words)

Words and Expressions

pandemic	/pænˈdemik/	n.	流行病
contention	/kənˈtenʃn/	n.	争论
patent	/ˈpæt（ə）nt/	n.	专利
skeptical	/ˈskeptikl/	adj.	怀疑的
elusive	/iˈluːsiv/	adj.	难懂的
frontier	/ˈfrʌntiə（r）/	n.	前沿
purification	/ˌpjʊərifiˈkeiʃn/	n.	提纯
identification	/aiˌdentifiˈkeiʃn/	n.	鉴定，识别
optional	/ˈɒpʃənl/	adj.	可选择的，随意的
toxicology	/ˌtɒksiˈkɒlədʒi/	n.	毒物学，毒理学
alleviate	/əˈliːvieit/	v.	减轻；缓和
consensus	/kənˈsensəs/	n.	一致；舆论
leverage	/ˈliːvəridʒ/	v.	利用
traction	/ˈtrækʃn/	n.	牵引
clinical efficacy		临床效果	

Proper Names

COVID-19	新冠肺炎
Compound Danshen Dripping Pill	复方丹参滴丸
HMPL-004	穿心莲提取物是一种作用于多靶点的口服植物药，用于治疗自身免疫性肠道疾病
Xuezhikang	血脂康胶囊，中成药名。由红曲组成。具有化浊降脂、活血化瘀、健脾消食的功效

After-reading Exercises

Task 1   Read the passage and choose the correct answer to each question.

(   ) 1. Which of the following statements is correct?

   A. The world medical professionals are stillunsure about TCM's efficacy

   B. The world medical professionals now accept TCM as curative for COVID-19

   C. The world has discovered the secrets of COVID-19

   D. Western medical communities do not deny the large strong trial data

(   ) 2. "off guard" from paragraph 2 means _____ .

   A. prepared   B. not prepared

   C. protected   D. not protected

(   ) 3. "Clinical protocol" from paragraph 2 can most probably defined as _____ .

   A. Clinical formality   B. Clinical treaty

   C. Clinical agreement   D. Clinical trial permission

(   ) 4. Which of the following statements is NOT true?

    A. Western medicine is based on science.

    B. TCM is based on practice.

    C. TCM often works as a mixture of components whose effect is easy to identify.

    D. Components in TCM work together to relieve certain symptoms.

( ) 5. What is the situation TCM is faced with?

    A. The western world is still skeptical about it.

    B. The western world is beginning to show interest in it.

    C. People are confident about TCM becoming popular.

    D. TCM has a disadvantage in treating chronic diseases.

Task 2   Translate the following sentences into Chinese.

1. In the midst of the still-unfolding novel coronavirus pandemic, traditional Chinese medicine (TCM) has once again become the bone of contention.

_____

2. While a set of Chinese patent drugs have proven effective in treating mildly symptomatic patients, Western medical communities are skeptical, citing a dearth of rigorous trial data to question their clinical efficacy.

_____

3. Faced with this new, elusive virus that caught the world off guard, major countries are all working on the scientific frontier to develop clinical protocols in the absence of a widely recognized vaccine.

_____

4. Western medicine is based on the science of pharmacology and toxicology while TCM is more empirically-based through a history of thousands of years.

_____

5. Chinese medicine has its uniqueness and advantages, especially in preventing and treating chronic diseases. It has a strong fit when we look at the macro trend of an aging population.

_____

Practical Writing

Company Profile

公司简介是对企业的介绍。这种介绍不是一句话带过，也不是长篇大论，是简单扼要的介绍公司的一段文字，让别人初步了解公司的基本情况。公司简介一般包括：公司概况、主要产品、公司文化（目标，理念，宗旨）等。

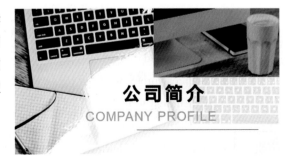

Sample

Pfizer

In 1849, cousins Charles Pfizer and Charles Erhart founded Charles Pfizer & Company in a red brick building in Brooklyn, NY.

We have a leading portfolio of products and medicines that support wellness and prevention, as well as treatment and cures for diseases across a broad range of therapeutic areas; and we have an industry-leading pipeline of promising new products that have the potential to challenge some of the most feared diseases of our time, like Alzheimer's disease and cancer.

Through working in partnership with everyone from patients to health care providers and managed care organizations to world governments and non-governmental organizations, our goal is to ensure that people everywhere have access to innovative treatments and quality health care.

公司简介常用词组及句型：

1. Co. Ltd：有限公司。

2. The company was founded by…：公司由…创立。

3. under one's leadership：在…的领导下。

4. adhere to the development strategy of…：坚持…的发展战略。

5. take …as the guide/ lead 以…为龙头/驱动。

6. operating model：经营模式。

7. The … system guided by … has been set up/ established：以……为指导的……的体系已建立。

8. The model got highly recognition of …, appreciating it as…：该模式得到了……的高度认可，被誉为……。

Task　Liu Lu is a manager's assistant in Yiling Pharmaceutical Company. Now he is going to write a company profile. Complete it with the information given below.

石家庄以岭制药有限公司是由中国工程院院士（Academician of the Chinese Academy of Engineering）吴以岭创办的国家重点高新技术企业（a national key high-tech enterprise）。在他的领导下，以岭药业始终坚持市场龙头、科技驱动的创新发展战略。为此，公司建立了"理论—临床—科研—产业—教学"五位一体（the five-in-one）的经营模式，也建立了以中医络病（Traditional Chinese Medicine collateral disease）理论创新为指导的新药开发创新技术体系。"五位一体"的经营模式得到了中华人民共和国科学技术部（the Ministry of Science and Technology of PRC）领导的高度肯定，被誉为"中医药科技成果产业化的开拓性工作"（the pioneering work in the industrialization of scientific and technological achievements in…）。

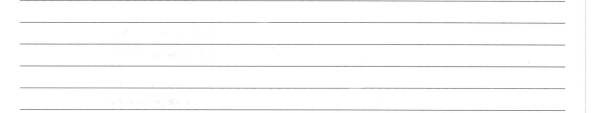

Grammar Tips

名词性从句包括主语从句、表语从句和宾语从句，因为这三个从句在句子中的功用相当于一个名词。名词性从句所用的关联词大抵相同，而且其前一般不用逗号。

Noun Clauses

从句类型	定义	关联词及注意事项
主语从句 Subject Clause	用作主语的从句	that（无意义，只连接）、whether（是否）、if（是否）从属连接；who、what、which 等疑问代词及 when、where、why、how 等疑问副词。连接代词和连接副词在句中既保留自己的疑问含义，又起连接作用。从句用陈述语序
	e. g. That we shall be late is certain. 　　　 Who he is doesn't concern me. 　　　 It is certain that we shall be late. （It 作形式主语）
表语从句 Predicative clause	用作表语的从句	引导表语从句的关联词与引导主语从句的关联词大都一样。从句用陈述语序
	e. g. His wish is to become a pharmacist.
宾语从句 Object clause	用作宾语的从句	引导宾语从句的关联词与引导主语从句的关联词大都一样。从句用陈述语序。时态要求：如果主句谓语动词是过去时态，则从句的时态要有相应的变化，也就是时态呼应，从句由现在时态变过去时态，由过去时态变为过去完成时态，将来时态变为过去将来时态，情态动词如为现在式，则应作相应改变。从句如为客观事实和真理，则不用改变
	e. g. I don't know if you can help me.

Task 1　Identify the Noun Clauses of each underlined italics part in the following sentences.

1. *What he did* is not yet known.　　　　　　　　　　　　_____

2. This is *what he meant*.　　　　　　　　　　　　_____

3. *Who he is* doesn't concern me.　　　　　　　　　　_____

4. The question is *how he did* it.　　　　　　　　　　_____

5. She saw *what food I bought*.　　　　　　　　　　_____

6. Do you know *who all these people are*?　　　　　_____

7. That's *where he lives*.　　　　　　　　　　　　　_____

8. I wonder *when he will come*.　　　　　　　　　　_____

9. She asked me *which I liked best*.　　　　　　　　_____

10. It is said *that he's got married*.　　　　　　　　_____

Task 2　Choose the best answer to complete each sentence.

(　) 1. Without his support, we wouldn't be _____ we are now.

　　　A.　how　　　　　　　　　　　B.　when

　　　C.　where　　　　　　　　　　D.　why

(　) 2. This is _____ my father has taught me——to always face difficulties and hope for the best.

　　　A.　how　　　　　　　　　　　B.　which

　　　C.　that　　　　　　　　　　　D.　what

(　) 3. She asked me _____ I had returned the books to the library.

    A. that   B. where

    C. whether   D. what

(　) 4. I don't know _____ .

    A. how to do   B. what I should do

    C. where should I go   D. when will he go

(　) 5. _____ he is still alive is a wonder.

    A. That   B. If

    C. Whether   D. Why

(　) 6. _____ they would support us was a problem.

    A. That   B. If

    C. Whether   D. It

(　) 7. He said he _____ like her.

    A. didn't   B. doesn't

    C. don't   D. won't

(　) 8. My problem is _____ I should ask him for help.

    A. if   B. whether

    C. that   D. what

(　) 9. He made it quite clear _____ he preferred to learn English.

    A. where   B. that

    C. when   D. which

(　) 10. He said _____ he couldn't tell you right away and _____ you wouldn't understand.

    A. that; how   B. that; /

    C. /; /   D. /;　that

Supplementary Reading

Lianhua Qingwen Medicine

Lianhua Qingwen medicine is a very common traditional Chinese medicine used for the treatment of cold and flu. Composed of 13 herbal components, it has shown curative effects on mild and common patients, especially in relieving fever, cough and fatigue. It can reduce the occurrence of deterioration and help patients test negative.

On April 14, 2020, Yiling Pharmaceutical announced that Yiling Pharmaceutical and its subsidiary Beijing Yiling Pharmaceutical had received the approval document of drug supplement application concerning the application for new indications of Lianhua Qingwen capsules and Lianhua Qingwen granules issued by National Medical Products Administration.

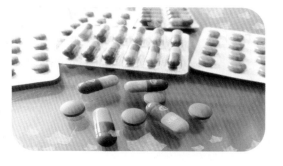

Lianhua Qingwen capsule and Lianhua Qingwen granules were approved to add "functional indications" to the originally approved indications: "In the conventional treatment of novel coronavirus pneumonia, it can be used for a light, common type of fever, cough, and fatigue", "Usage and dosage" increased "COVID-19 light, normal treatment for 7-10 days" and so on.

In this domestic epidemic, Lianhua Qingwen capsules (granules) became the most frequently recommended Chinese patent medicine for COVID-19. In the fourth to the seventh edition of the novel pneumonia diagnosis and treatment scheme infected by coronavirus published by National Health Commission of the People's Republic of China and National Administration of Traditional Chinese Medicine, it is recommended to take the Chinese patent medicine Lianhua Qingwen capsule (granule) for the prevention and treatment of patients with fatigue and fever during the medical observation period.

The efficacy of the Lianhua Qingwen capsule (granule) in the treatment of COVID-19 has been confirmed by basic experiments and clinical studies. Zhong Nanshan's team recently published a paper entitled "The antiviral and anti-inflammatory effect of the antipyretic plague on novel coronavirus" in the international journal "Pharmacology Research", which was the first basic research article of effective Chinese patent medicine against SARS-Cov-2. In this study, it was found that Lianhua Qingwen could significantly inhibit the replication of novel coronavirus in cells, and the expression of virus particles in cells was significantly reduced after the treatment of coronavirus.

It is reported that this approval is in the originally approved indications based on the addition of the "COVID-19 light, ordinary type" of the new indications. At the same time, the new batch of prescription drug specifications did not deny the original non-prescription drug positioning.

Up to now, Lianhua Qingwen capsules have been registered in Hong Kong (SAR of China), Macao (SAR of China), Brazil, Indonesia, Canada, Mozambique, Romania and other places as "Chinese patent medicine", "medicine", "plant medicine" and "natural health products", and have been approved for marketing.

(417 words)

After-reading Exercises

Task Decide whether the following statements are true (T) or false (F) according to the text.

(   ) 1. Lianhua Qingwen capsule can be effective on fatally sick patients.

(   ) 2. Lianhua Qingwen medicine got the permission from State Drug Administration on April 14, 2020.

(   ) 3. The state administration of TCM suggested that patients take Lianhua Qingwen capsule for symptoms of fatigue and fever during medical observation.

(   ) 4. Whether Lianhua Qingwen capsule is effective is to be discussed for COVID-19.

(   ) 5. Some countries and areas in the world have already permitted Lianhua Qingwen capsule to go to their market.

Vocabulary Tips

Prefix "cardi-/ cardio-"：心。

Example：cardiovascular 心血管的；cardiac 心脏的；carditis 心脏炎；cardiogram 心动图；electrocardiogram 心电图。

Prefix "pan-"：总，全，泛。

Example：pandemic 大范围传染的；panacea 万能药；panorama 全景；pantheism 泛神论。

Root "toxic-"：有毒的，与毒相关的。

Example：toxicity 毒性；toxicology 毒理学；toxicant 有毒物，毒药；toxicological 毒物学的；detoxication 解毒。

Task　Complete the sentences with the given words.

electrocardiogram	cardiac	panacea	panorama	toxicity

1. The man was suffering from _____ weakness.

2. There is a superb _____ of the mountains from the hotel.

3. To measure the heart rate, for instance, the shirt contains a pair of non-sticky sensors（非粘贴式传感器）that can produce a simplified _____.

4. Every chemical has _____, but it's all in the dose.

5. But cardiac experts warned alcohol was not a _____ for good heart health.

Proverbs and Sayings

◇Patience is the plaster for all sores.

　　耐心是最好的药方。

◇A disease known is half cured.

　　明确诊断，治好一半。

◇If the pills were pleasant, they would not want gilding.

　　药丸若好吃，毋需果糖衣。

题库

PPT

Unit 5

Drug Development

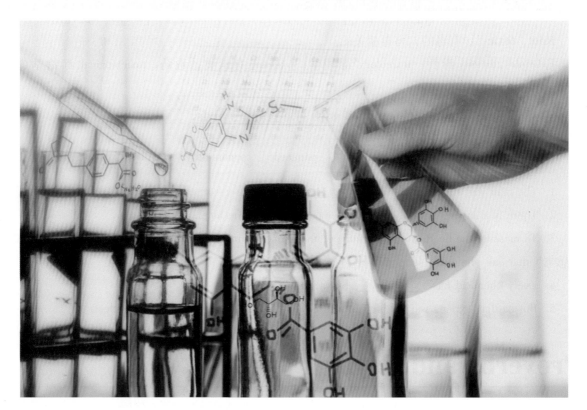

Unit Objectives

After studying this unit, you are expected to:

· master the vocabulary and technical terms related to drug development;

· understand the drug development process and the discovery of artemisinin;

· know attributive clause correctly.

And you should learn how to:

· communicate with others about the development of some great drugs;

· write a poster.

Introduction

医药大学堂
WWW.YIYADDXT.COM

Introduction

Drug development is the process of bringing a new pharmaceutical drug to the market once a lead compound has been identified through the process of drug discovery. It includes preclinical research on microorganisms and animals, filing for regulatory status, such as via the United States Food and Drug Administration for an investigational new drug to initiate clinical trials on humans, and may include the step of obtaining regulatory approval with a new drug application to market the drug.

There are five critical steps in the U. S. drug development process, and they are as follows:

Step 1: Discovery and Development.

Step 2: Preclinical Research.

Step 3: Clinical Research.

Step 4: FDA Review.

Step 5: FDA Post-Market Safety Monitoring.

Warming-up

Task　Work in groups. Match the pictures to the proper statements. Then check your answers with your partner.

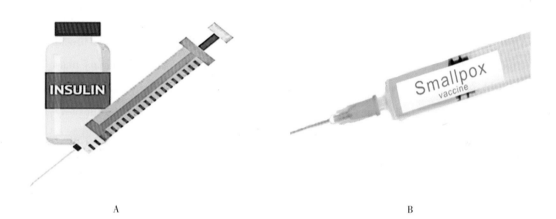

A

B

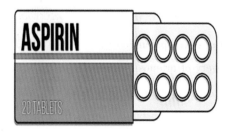

C

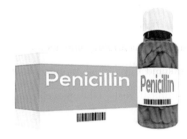

D

(　) 1. It is effective against many bacterial infections caused by staphylococci and streptococci.

(　) 2. It regulates the metabolism of carbohydrates, fats and protein by promoting the absorption of glucose from the blood into liver, fat and skeletal muscle cells.

(　) 3. From 1958 to 1977, the World Health Organization conducted a global vaccination campaign that eradicated smallpox, making it the only human disease to be eradicated.

( ) 4. It is used to reduce fever and relieve mild to moderate pain from conditions such as muscle aches, toothaches, common cold, and headaches.

Reading A

The Drug Development Process

Across the drug industry there are several mandated processes that must be undergone before the final sale of a drug can begin on the market. One of the most important phases for a drug overall is its Food and Drug Administration (FDA) approval. As such this article looks at the five comprehensive phases the FDA outlines for a successful drug development process with the fourth phase being the FDA's review.

Step 1: Discovery and Development

Each drug begins with discovery and development in a lab. Pharma companies spend millions of dollars on research and development that includes scientific study and development of drugs for new innovation. Funding can come from several areas including government, grants, and revenues.

Step 2: Preclinical Research

Once a drug discovery has been made it must go through both preclinical and clinical research with supporting reports tied to its review process. Preclinical research is a basic preliminary phase that involves testing the drug on animals and basic testing for safety flags. Usually, preclinical studies are not very large. However, these studies must provide detailed information on dosing and toxicity levels. After preclinical testing, researchers review their findings and decide whether the drug should be tested in people.

Step 3: Clinical Research

Clinical research can be one of the most important steps in a drug's development. If a drug is cleared from preclinical trials, it moves on to clinical testing which involves human trials. Drug companies and the FDA have specific standards for clinical trials which include the professionals involved in the scientific testing, the selection criteria of the humans being tested, the setting in

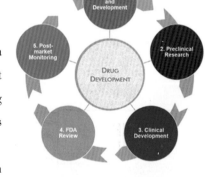

which the clinical tests take place, and more. Clinical trial registration is also required and heavily followed by pharma professionals across the sector. Clinical trials follow a typical series from early, small-scale, phase 1 studies to late-stage, large scale, phase 3 studies.

Step 4: FDA Review

The Food and Drug Administration is one of the primary regulators involved in all aspects of the drug market. The high standards for drug approval in the U. S. often lead drug development testing in the first three phases to last for approximately 10 to 15 years before approval. In phase four, companies submit fully documented research and findings to the FDA for review. If a submission is accepted, the FDA will provide a response within 6 to 10 months.

Step 5: FDA Post-Market Safety Monitoring

There are several aspects of post-approval safety monitoring for a marketed drug. The FDA monitors all types of drug advertising for accuracy. It also monitors complaints and problems associated with a drug. As such it has the power to limit drug sales and offer warnings. In general, the FDA also does routine manufacturing inspections. Furthermore, the FDA is involved in the patent protections and generic drug transitions of all drugs.

(473 words)

Reading A
Words and
Expressions

Words and Expressions			
mandate	/'mændeit/	vt.	授权；托管
undergo	/ˌʌndə'gəʊ/	vt.	经历，经受
approval	/ə'pruːvl/	n.	批准；认可
pharma	/'fɑːmə/	n.	制药公司
revenue	/'revənjuː/	n.	税收收入；财政收入
preclinical	/priː'klinik(ə)l/	adj.	临床前的
dosing	/'dəʊsiŋ/	n.	定量给料，配量
toxicity	/tɒk'sisəti/	n.	毒性
criteria	/krai'tiəriə/	n.	标准，条件
submit	/səb'mit/	vt.	呈递；提交
inspection	/in'spekʃn/	n.	视察，检查
transition	/træn'ziʃn/	n.	过渡；转变
preclinical research		临床前研究	
clinical research		临床研究	
human trial		人体试验	
clinical trial registration		临床试验注册	
patent protection		专利保护	
generic drug		仿制药	

📖 Notes

1. Across the drug industry there are several mandated processes that must be undergone before the final sale of a drug can begin on the market.

在整个制药行业，药品最终销售开始上市之前，必须经过若干法定流程。

"across" 意为 "在…各处；遍及"。

e. g. Her family is scattered across the country.

她家中的人散居全国各地。

e. g. This view is common across all sections of the community.

该社群所有阶层的人普遍持有这种看法。

2. Pharma companies spend millions of dollars on research and development that includes scientific study and development of drugs for new innovation.

制药公司花费数百万美元进行研发，包括科学研究和开发药物以进行新的创新。

"spend sth. on sth. /(on) doing sth." 意为 "用，花（钱）"。

医药大学堂
www.yiyaodxt.com

e. g. The company has spent thousands of pounds updating their computer systems.

公司花了几千英镑更新计算机系统。

"that includes scientific study and development of drugs for new innovation" 为 that 引导的定语从句，修饰先行词 research and development。

3. Once a drug discovery has been made it must go through both preclinical and clinical research with supporting reports tied to its review process.

一旦一种药物被发现，它必须经过临床前和临床研究，并有与审查过程相关的支持报告。

"go through" 意为 "通过；经历"。

e. g. He's amazingly cheerful considering all he's had to go through.

经历了种种磨难，他还那么乐观，令人惊叹。

"tied to its review process" 过去分词短语作定语，相当于定语从句 "which are tied to its review process"。

4. If a drug is cleared from preclinical trials, it moves on to clinical testing which involves human trials.

如果一种药物通过了临床前试验，它就会进入涉及人体试验的临床试验。

"clear" 意为 "批准；准许；得到许可"。

e. g. His appointment had been cleared by the board.

他的任命已由董事会批准。

5. Drug companies and the FDA have specific standards for clinical trials which include the professionals involved in the scientific testing, the selection criteria of the humans being tested, the setting in which the clinical tests take place, and more.

制药公司和 FDA 有具体的临床试验标准，其中包括参与科学测试的专业人员、被检人员的选择标准、进行临床试验的环境等。

"involve in" 意为 "参与；涉及"。

e. g. Insulin resistance as the important virulence factor involve in the pathogenesis of both diabetes and heart or brain vascular disease.

胰岛素抵抗是心脑血管疾病和糖尿病的重要致病因子，与二者的发生发展密切相关。

6. The high standards for drug approval in the U. S. often lead drug development testing in the first three phases to last for approximately 10 to 15 years before approval.

美国高标准的药品审批要求通常会导致药物研发测试的前三个阶段要持续大约 10 到 15 年才能获得批准。

"lead to" 意为 "致使；导致"。

e. g. Salt intake may lead to raised blood pressure in susceptible adults.

盐的摄入可能导致易患病的成年人血压升高。

After-reading Exercises

Task 1 Answer the following questions according to the text.

1. What are the five comprehensive phases the FDA outlines for a successful drug development

process?

_____

2. Where does the funding for drug development come from?

_____

3. What is the preclinical research involved in?

_____

4. When can a drug move on to clinical testing which involves human trials?

_____

5. How long will the FDA provide a response if a submission is accepted?

_____

Task 2　Match the words（1-10）to the Chinese meanings（a-j）.

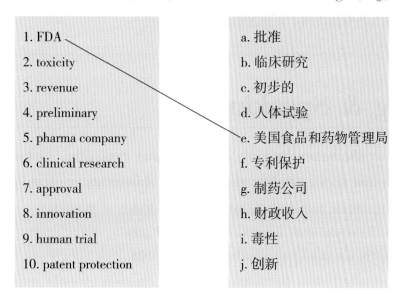

1. FDA
2. toxicity
3. revenue
4. preliminary
5. pharma company
6. clinical research
7. approval
8. innovation
9. human trial
10. patent protection

a. 批准
b. 临床研究
c. 初步的
d. 人体试验
e. 美国食品和药物管理局
f. 专利保护
g. 制药公司
h. 财政收入
i. 毒性
j. 创新

Task 3　Fill in each blank with the proper form of the word or phrase given in brackets.

1. Across the drug industry there are several _____ processes that must be undergone before the final sale of a drug can begin on the market.（mandate）

2. Preclinical research is a basic preliminary phase that involves _____ the drug on animals and basic testing for safety flags.（test）

3. If a drug is _____ from preclinical trials, it moves on to clinical testing which involves human trials.（clear）

4. Clinical trial registration is also required and heavily _____ by pharma professionals across the sector.（follow）

5. There are several aspects of post-approval safety _____ for a marketed drug.（monitor）

Task 4　Translate the following sentences into English using the words or phrases you have learned in this unit.

1. 每种药物都是从实验室的发现和开发开始。（begin with）

_____

2. 临床试验遵循一系列的研究流程，从早期、小规模、第一阶段研究到晚期、大规模、第三阶段研究。（follow）

_____

3. 美国食品和药物管理局是药品市场各个方面的主要监管机构之一。（involve）

_____

4. 如果申请被接受，FDA 将在 6 到 10 个月内给出答复。（provide a response）

_____

5. FDA 监控所有类型的药物广告的真实性。（monitor）

_____

Listening & Speaking

Listening &
Speaking
Task 1

Task 1　Two pharmacy students are discussing Penicillin. Listen to the conversation and decide whether the following statements are true(T) or false(F).

Which is One of the Most Powerful Killers of Bacteria?

(　) 1. Penicillin is one of the most powerful killers of virus.

(　) 2. Penicillin was discovered quite by accident in 1928.

(　) 3. One evening Fleming placed a cover on one of the plates, when he came the next morning he saw some blue-green mould had grown on the plate during the night.

(　) 4. If Fleming had not noticed that small area of mould on his plate, he would not have discovered the powerful antibiotic.

(　) 5. It was not until 1940 that penicillin was reported a safe drug for use on humans.

📖 **Notes**

1. Fleming put some of the mould together with more bacteria of the same kind, the germs were also destroyed.

弗莱明把一些霉菌和更多相同种类的细菌放在一起，细菌也被摧毁了。

"together with" 意为 "和；连同"。

e. g. I switched to traditional medicine and all the hives disappeared, together with my itching.

我转而服用传统药物，我的荨麻疹和瘙痒都消失了。

2. If Fleming had not noticed that small area of mould on his plate, he would not have discovered this powerful antibiotic.

如果弗莱明没有注意到他的盘子里那小块霉菌，他就不会发现这种强大的抗生素。

3. It was reported a safe drug for use on humans and made available to doctors until 1941.

直到 1941 年，它才被报道是可用于人类的安全药物，并可供医生使用。

"make available to" 意为 "可供使用；向……提供"。

e. g. We are here to make available to you, as best we can, that expertise.

我们任务就是尽最大努力使你们能够获得那些专门知识。

Task 2　After Professor Chen's lecture, Li Jing is asking him questions on drug development. Listen to the conversation and answer the following questions.

What is Critical for Commercial Success in Drug Development?

(　) 1. What does "drug candidate" mean?

  A. The end-product of the discovery phase

  B. The end-product of the preclinical phase

  C. The end-product of the clinical phase

  D. Not mentioned

(　) 2. What is critical for commercial success in drug development?

  A. Price   B. Quality

  C. Efficiency   D. Marketing

(　) 3. Drug development accounts for about _____ of the total R&D costs.

  A. 3/4   B. 1/4

  C. 1/3   D. 2/3

(　) 4. _____ in development is also an important factor in determining sales revenue.

  A. Cost   B. Speed

  C. Both A and B   D. Not mentioned

(　) 5. Decide the following statements, which one is correct?

  A. Drug development means transforming a drug candidate to an approved product

  B. The cost per project is the greatest in the development phase

  C. Once the patent expires, generic competition sharply reduces sales revenue

  D. Keeping the quality under control is a major concern for management

📖 Notes

1. Drug development accounts for about two-thirds of the total R&D costs.

药物开发约占研发总成本的三分之二。

"accounts for" 意为 "占…比例"。

e. g. While malaria accounts for 40 percent of all child deaths in the country, all of the population of the DRC is vulnerable to the disease.

尽管因疟疾而死亡儿童人数占该国总死亡人数的 40%，但该国的成年人口也容易患上这种病。

2. The cost per project is very much greater in the development phase, and increases sharply as the project moves into the later phases of clinical development.

每个项目的成本在开发阶段就比较大，随着项目进入临床开发后期阶段，其成本会急剧增加。

Listening &
Speaking
Task 3

Task 3 The following passage is about methods of exploring vaccine candidates. Listen carefully and fill in the blanks with what you hear.

Technology is enabling new methods of exploring vaccine candidates for trial, but there are already a few tried and tested ways to make them. In all of them, scientists try to stimulate the body's _____1_____ system to combat _____2_____ pathogen. That's commonly done by creating something so similar to the pathogen that the body begins to create _____3_____ to fight off the real thing. The most common way of doing this is to make what's called _____4_____ vaccines-those that are made of weaker strains of the actual pathogen. Reared on animal cells outside of human bodies, they are then extracted and _____5_____ in a single tiny dose. Vaccines for measles and tuberculosis are created in this way.

Task 4 Work in groups, try to discuss the topic of "Penicillin". Practice with your partner according to what you hear in the Listening part.

Partner A	Partner B
Greet.	Greet and show an interest in Penicillin.
Introduce Dr. Alexander Fleming.	How was penicillin discovered by accident?
Tell the story in 1928.	Value Fleming's work greatly.
Explain further (widely used in 1941).	Show the appreciation.

Reading B

Artemisinin: Anti-malarial Drugs in China

Discovered by Youyou Tu, one of the 2015 Nobel Prize winners in Physiology or Medicine, together with many other Chinese scientists, artemisinin, artemether and artesunate, as well as other artemisinins, have brought the global anti-malarial treatment to a new era, saving millions of lives all around the world for the past 40 years.

In the late 1960s and 1970s, Tu was the head of an antimalarial research group, she led her group of young scholars in the extraction and isolation of constituents with possible antimalarial activities from Chinese herbs. During the first stage of this research, her group investigated more than 2,000 Chinese herb preparations and identified 640 recipes that might have some antimalarial activities. More than 380 extracts, obtained from some 200 Chinese herbs, and including extracts from *Artemisia annua* L. , were tested against a rodent malaria model. However, progress was not smooth and no significant results were obtained at first.

The turning point came when an *Artemisia* extract showed a promising degree of inhibition against parasite growth, consistent with activity which had been reported for this species in *A Handbook of Prescriptions for Emergencies* by Ge Hong (Jin Dynasty, 284-346 A. D.). Tu brilliantly modified the extraction technique to perform it at low temperature, rather than using heating, as was conventional. And she found

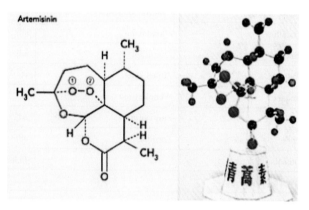

that the most effective preparation came from the leaves of *Artemisia annua* L. , as evidenced by its significant inhibition of mouse malaria *P. berghei*. Tu was able to separate the extract into an acidic portion, which contained no antimalarial activity, and a neutral extract, which exhibited both reduced toxicity and improved antimalarial activity.

After their first human experiments, Tu and her team went to Hainan to verify the efficacy of the extract clinically, and carried out antimalarial trails with patients infected with both *P. vivax* and *P. falciparum*. These clinical trials produced encouraging feedback, achieving a rapid disappearance of fever and parasites from the blood as compared with the control group using chloroquine. Tu next investigated the isolation and purification of the active component from *Artemisia annua* L. Eventually, in 1972, her team identified a colorless crystalline substance with a molecular weight of 282 Da, a molecular formula of $C_{15}H_{22}O_5$ and a melting point of 156-157°C, as the active principal and named it "Qinghaosu". However, because of the prevailing environment, not many papers concerning Qinghaosu were published.

Plasmodium falciparum has been a life-threatening disease for thousands of years and still threatens millions of lives every year in many parts of the world, particularly in Africa. After a failed international attempt to eradicate malaria in the 1950s, the disease rebounded. Artemisinin was a new antimalarial agent with a totally different chemical structure and a higher efficacy, as compared with the conventional drugs against which resistance has been acquired and the successful application of artemisinin and its derivatives for treating several thousand malaria patients in China attracted worldwide attention in the 1980s. The discovery of artemisinin has since been recognized as a significant milestone in the human journey towards conquering malaria.

(510 words)

Words and Expressions

physiology	/ˌfizi'ɒlədʒi/	n.	生理学；生理机能
artemisinin	/ˌɑːti'miːsinin/	n.	青蒿素（抗疟药）
antimalarial	/ˌæntiməˈleəriəl/	adj.	［药］抗疟疾的
extraction	/ikˈstrækʃn/	n.	取出；抽出；抽出物
rodent	/ˈrəʊdnt/	n.	啮齿目动物

续表

inhibition	/ˌinhiˈbiʃn/	n.	抑制；压抑
parasite	/ˈpærəsait/	n.	寄生虫；食客
chloroquine	/ˈklɔːrə(ʊ)kwiːn/	n.	[药] 氯喹
crystalline	/ˈkristəlain/	adj.	透明的；水晶般的
principal	/ˈprinsəpl/	adj.	主要的
eradicate	/iˈrædikeit/	vt.	根除，根绝；消灭
conquer	/ˈkɒŋkə(r)/	vt.	战胜，征服；攻克
prevailing	/priˈveiliŋ/	adj.	流行的；盛行很广的
acidic	/əˈsidik/	adj.	酸的，酸性的
antimalarial activity		抗疟活性	
Proper Names			
Artemisiaannua L.		黄花蒿	
P. berghei		伯氏鼠疟原虫	
P. vivax		间日疟原虫	
P. falciparum		恶性疟原虫	

After-reading Exercises

Task 1　Read the passage and choose the correct answer to each question.

(　) 1. For her discoveries, Tu received the Nobel Prize for Physiology or Medicine _____ .

A. in 1972　　　　　　　　B. in 1980

C. in 2011　　　　　　　　D. in 2015

(　) 2. Which of the followinghas brought the global anti-malarial treatment to a new era?

A. Artemisinin　　　　　　B. Artemether

C. Artesunate　　　　　　D. A, B and C

(　) 3. The author of *A Handbook of Prescriptions for Emergencies* is _____ .

A. Zhang Zhongjing　　　　B. Ge Hong

C. Sun Simiao　　　　　　D. Zhu Danxi

(　) 4. The molecular formula of "Qinghaosu" is _____ .

A. $C_{15}H_{22}O_5$　　　　　　B. $C_{15}H_{21}O_5$

C. $C_{16}H_{22}O_5$　　　　　　D. $C_{13}H_{22}O_5$

(　) 5. Which of the following has been a life-threatening disease for thousands of years?

A. *P. berghei*　　　　　　B. *P. vivax*

C. *P. falciparum*　　　　　D. *Artemisia annua* L.

Task 2　Translate the following sentences into Chinese.

1. During the first stage of this research, her group investigated more than 2,000 Chinese herb preparations and identified 640 recipes that might have some antimalarial activities.

_____

2. Tu brilliantly modified the extraction technique to perform it at low temperature, rather than using

heating, as was conventional.

3. Tu was able to separate the extract into an acidic portion, which contained no antimalarial activity, and a neutral extract, which exhibited both reduced toxicity and improved antimalarial activity.

4. *Plasmodium falciparum* has been a life-threatening disease for thousands of years and still threatens millions of lives every year in many parts of the world, particularly in Africa.

5. The discovery of artemisinin has since been recognized as a significant milestone in the human journey towards conquering malaria.

Practical Writing

Posters

海报是我们日常生活中极为常见、告知公众有关信息的招贴，主要用于宣传电影、戏剧、比赛、文艺演出等活动。海报由标题、正文和落款三部分构成。

标题：居于海报正上方，用简洁、引人注目的语言概括主题。正文：是对海报标题的具体描述，常用一些鼓动性较强的语句来吸引读者的注意力，表现形式有说明式、美术设计式、图表式等。落款：注明主办单位及发布海报的日期。

The Last Lecture
Life lessons in 60 minutes

Office of Student Life invites
Professor Aaron Cassill
to deliver the inaugural
UTSA Last Lecture.

November 5ᵗʰ @ 7:00 pm
Retama Auditorium
University Center

For more info.
210-458-7967

Sample

Free Lectures on
"Keeping Them Safe: A Focus on Opioid Use in Pregnancy and Pregnancy Outcomes"
By Dr. Rotimi Orisatoki
From 12:00 p.m. to 1:00 p.m.
Tuesday, Feb. 25ᵗʰ, 2020
Hurlburt Auditorium
604-682-2344

Foreign Language College
Feb. 20ᵗʰ, 2020

海报通常包含以下项目。
标题：Title；
目的：Purpose；

时间：Time；

地点：Place；

联系方式：Contact information；

主办单位：Organizer。

Task Suppose you are the President of the Student Union of a medical college, Li Jing. Your college is going to hold a Medical English Corner. On behalf of the Student Union, please design an English poster and post it on your college's English website to invite students to participate.

时间：10 月 13 日晚 6：00 – 8：00

地点：英语公园

联系方式：13974810582

Join Our Medical English Corner

———————————

Come and join us!

Here you can

talk to foreign medical professionals

———————————
———————————

make new friends

———————————
———————————
———————————
———————————

Students' Union

Oct. 10th, 2020

Grammar Tips

定语从句是由关系代词和关系副词引导的从句，其作用是作定语修饰主句的某个名词性成分，定语从句分为限制性和非限制性从句两种。定语从句的基本结构为：先行词 + 关系代词或关系副词 + 从句本身。

Attributive Clauses

例句	语法成分	功能
关系代词		
who/that　Do you know the man who/that is standing by the window?	主语	指人

续表

	例句	语法成分	功能
whom/that	The man whom/that you spoke to just now is my friend.	宾语	指人
which/that	Don't forget to bring the book which/that the teacher gave you the other day.	宾语	指物
whose	1. The patients whose temperature isn't normal are in the wards. 2. The book whose cover is red is an English book.	定语	指人或物
that	She is no longer the girl that she was before she was married.	表语	指人
as	As we all know, the earth is round.	主语或宾语	
关系副词			
when	He came at a time when we needed help.	状语	时间
where	We know the place where our teacher lives.	状语	地点
why	Do you know the reason why he was so happy?	状语	原因

Task 1   Complete the following sentences with appropriate relative pronouns or adverbs.

1. This is the best factory _____ we visited last year.

2. The games _____ the young men competed in were difficult.

3. Please pass me the dictionary _____ cover is red.

4. The comrade _____ is speaking at the meeting is my teacher.

5. He asked us to watch carefully everything _____ he did in class.

6. I'll visit the professor tomorrow, _____ he will be back from Shanghai.

7. The city _____ my mother grew up is not far from here.

8. Our teacher lives in the house _____ door faces to the north.

9. Wrestling is a sport in _____ people easily get hurt.

10. Is there anything _____ I can do for you, sir?

Task 2   Choose the best answer to complete each sentence.

(   ) 1. His parents wouldn't let him marry anyone _____ family was poor.

     A. of whom   B. whom

     C. of whose   D. whose

(   ) 2. She heard a terrible noise, _____ brought her heart into her mouth.

     A. it   B. which

     C. this   D. that

(   ) 3. In the dark street, there wasn't a single person _____ she could turn for help.

     A. that   B. who

     C. from whom   D. to whom

(   ) 4. The weather turned out to be very good, _____ was more than we could expect.

     A. what   B. which

     C. that   D. it

(   ) 5. After living in Pairs for fifty years he returned to the small town _____ he grew up as a child.

     A. which   B. where

C. that D. when

( ) 6. Carol said the work would be done by October, _____ personally I doubt very much.

    A. it B. that

    C. when D. which

( ) 7. Dorothy was always speaking highly of her role in the play, _____, of course, made the others unhappy.

    A. who B. which

    C. this D. what

( ) 8. Whenever I met him, _____ was fairly often, I like his sweet and hopeful smile.

    A. what B. which

    C. that D. when

( ) 9. _____ has already been pointed out, grammar is not a set of dead rules.

    A. As B. It

    C. That D. Which

( ) 10. I had neither a raincoat nor an umbrella. _____ I got wet through.

    A. It's the reason B. That's why

    C. There's why D. It's how

Supplementary Reading

Tu Youyou: Chinese Scientist and Phytochemist

Tu Youyou, (born December 30, 1930, Ningbo, Zhejiang province, China), Chinese scientist and phytochemist known for her isolation and study of the antimalarial substance *qinghaosu*, later known as artemisinin, one of the world's most-effective malaria-fighting drugs. For her discoveries, Tu received the 2015 Nobel Prize for Physiology or Medicine (shared with Irish-born American parasitologist William Campbell and Japanese microbiologist Satoshi ōmura).

Tu studied at the department of pharmaceutics of Beijing Medical College. After earning a degree there in 1955, she was chosen to join the Institute of Materia Medica at the Academy of Traditional Chinese Medicine (later the China Academy of Chinese Medical Sciences). From 1959 to 1962, she participated in a full-time training course in the use of traditional Chinese medicine that was geared toward researchers with knowledge of Western medicine. The course provided a foundation for her later application of traditional Chinese medical knowledge to modern drug discovery.

In 1967, during the Vietnam War (1955-1975), Tu was appointed to lead Project 523, Tu and her team of researchers began by identifying plants with supposed activity against malaria on the basis of information from folk medicine and remedies described in ancient Chinese medical texts. Her team identified some 640 plants and more than 2,000 remedies with potential antimalarial activity and subsequently tested 380 extracts from about 200 of the plant species for their ability to rid malaria-causing *Plasmodium* parasites from the blood of infected mice. An extract obtained from the sweet wormwood plant (*qinghao*), *Artemisia annua*, showed particular promise. In 1971, after refining the extraction process, Tu and colleagues successfully isolated a nontoxic extract from sweet wormwood that effectively eliminated *Plasmodium* parasites from mice and monkeys. Clinical studies were soon thereafter carried out in malaria patients, in whom sweet wormwood extracts were found to quickly lower fever and reduce parasite levels in the blood. In 1972 Tu and colleagues isolated the active compound in the extracts, which they named *qinghaosu*, or artemisinin.

Although Tu had relied on information from ancient texts, the works said little about the plant known as *qinghao*, and many of her team's early attempts to reproduce their initial findings on the plant's antimalarial activity failed. Eventually, however, Tu discovered that the leaves of sweet wormwood contain artemisinin and that the compound is extracted optimally at relatively low temperatures. Tu initially was prevented from publishing her

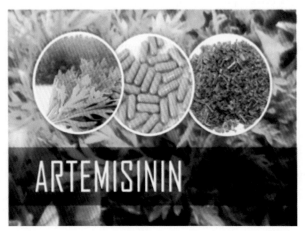

team's findings, because of restrictions on the publication of scientific information that were in place in China at the time. The work finally reached international audiences, to wide acclaim, in the early 1980s. In the early 2000s, the World Health Organization recommended the use of artemisinin-based combination drug therapies as first-line treatment for malaria.

Tu continued to investigate artemisinin and developed a second antimalarial compound, dihydroartemisinin, which is a bioactive artemisinin metabolite. In 2011 she received the Lasker-DeBakey Clinical Medical Research Award for her contributions to the discovery of artemisinin.

(487 words)

After-reading Exercises

Task　Decide whether the following statements are true (T) or false (F) according to the text.

(　　) 1. Tu Youyou is a Chinese scientist and phytochemist known for her isolation and study of the antimalarial substance *qinghaosu*, later known as artemisinin.

(　　) 2. Tu studied at the department of pharmaceutics of Beijing Medical College and earned a degree there in 1958.

(　　) 3. In 1967, during the Vietnam War (1954-1975), Tu was appointed to lead Project 532.

(　　) 4. In the early 2000s, the World Health Organization recommended the use of artemisinin-based combination drug therapies as first-line treatment for malaria.

(　　) 5. In 2011 she received Nobel Prize for Physiology or Medicine for her contributions to the discovery of artemisinin.

Vocabulary Tips

Prefix "anti-"：反对，相反，防止。

Example：antipathy 反感（anti＋pathy 感情）；antibacterial 抗菌的；antibody 抗体（anti＋body 身体）；anticontagious 防止传染的；anti-ageing 防衰老的；antigas 防毒气的；antifat 防止肥胖的。

Prefix "para-"：旁、靠近、外，辅助、副。

Example：parasite 寄生虫（site 食，在他体旁寄食者）；parabiosphere 外生物圈的；para-appendicitis 阑尾旁组织炎；paratyphoid 副伤寒；paramedical 医疗辅助工作的。

Task　Complete the sentences with the given words.

parasite　　antibody　　anti-ageing　　paramedical　　antibacterial

1. At the same time, some drugs are also known to have _____ properties——again, in "lower" animals.

2. Technicians and pharmacists are _____ personnel.

3. This helps get rid of _____ that produce some of the toxins in our body.

4. Rain water makes excellent soft washwater, but needs _____ treatment.

5. An _____ is an immune system protein that helps seek and destroy invaders like viruses and bacteria.

Proverbs and Sayings

◇Wherever the art of Medicine is loved, there is also a love of Humanity.

哪里有人爱医学艺术，哪里就有人爱人性。

◇In nothing do men more nearly approach the gods than in giving health to men.

没有什么比给予人健康更接近神的了。

◇Wear the white coat with dignity and pride-it is an honor and privilege to get to serve the public as a physician.

带着尊严和自豪穿上白大褂——作为一名医生为公众服务是一种荣誉和特权。

题库

医药大学堂
WWW.YIYADDXT.COM

Unit **6**

New Drug Application

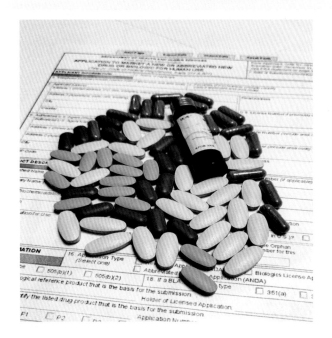

Unit Objectives

After studying this unit, you are expected to:

· master the vocabulary and technical terms related to New Drug Application;

· understand the United State New Drug Application and Chinese registration routes of imported drugs;

· know adverbial clause correctly.

And you should learn how to:

· communicate with pharmacists to buy drugs on a prescription or without a prescription;

· write an E-mail.

Introduction

New drugs are regulated and controlled in countries all over the world. A new drug application must be approved before a new drug can be marketed. In the United States, the FDA, which approves new drug applications, is the top law enforcement agency specializing in food and drug administration. Known as the "patron saint of America's Health" the FDA is known for its high standards and rigorous approval process.

Many other countries promote and monitor the safety of their own products by seeking and receiving FDA assistance.

In China, NMPA is the agency that approves new drug applications. NMPA is working on new measures to accelerate China's drug-regulation process and make it more rigorous, in line with international standards. "China could eventually develop a drug review and approval process that is faster and superior to countries in the West." According to a former pharmaceutical industry executive, George Baeder who is now a director of China Global Insight, a California-based think tank.

Warming-up

Task Which of the following products require FDA approval? Work in groups. Match the pictures with the proper statements. Then check your answers with your partner.

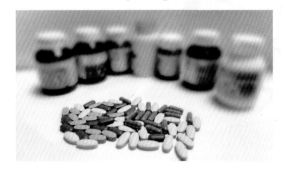

A

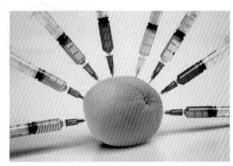

B

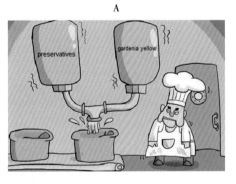

C

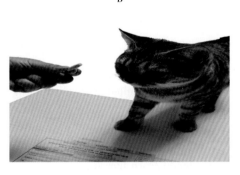

D

(　) 1. FDA approves food additives in food for people. Although FDA does not have premarket approval of food products, it has the authority to approve certain ingredients before they are used in foods. Those include food additives.

(　) 2. FDA approves color additives used in FDA-regulated products. This includes those used in food (including animal food), dietary supplements, drugs, cosmetics, and some medical devices.

(　) 3. FDA approves animal drugs and approves food additives for use in food for animals. FDA is responsible for approving drugs for animals, including pets, livestock, and poultry.

(　) 4. FDA approves new drugs and biologics. New drugs and certain biologics must be proven safe and effective to FDA's satisfaction before companies can market them in interstate commerce.

Reading A

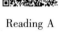

New Drug Application

For decades, the regulation and control of new drugs in the United States have been based on the New Drug Application (NDA). Since 1938, every new drug has been the subject of an approved NDA before U. S. commercialization.

What Is a New Drug Application (NDA)?

A new drug application (NDA) is a comprehensive document that must be submitted to the U. S. Food and Drug Administration (FDA) in order to request approval for marketing a new drug in the United States. It is the vehicle through which drug sponsors formally propose that the FDA approve a new pharmaceutical for sale and marketing in the U. S. The data gathered during the animal studies and human clinical trials of an Investigational New Drug (IND) become part of the NDA.

How New Drug Applications Work?

The filing of an NDA represents an important milestone in the life of a new drug and is closely watched by investors. Once the NDA has been submitted, the likelihood of that drug receiving FDA approval is usually very high. Accordingly, companies that file NDAs often see their share prices appreciate even before their response from the FDA is obtained.

Yet, reaching the NDA stage is far from easy. Each NDA document must contain 15 sections containing detailed experimental evidence (including both animal and human studies) . The document must extensively demonstrate the proposed drug's pharmacology, toxicology, and dosage requirements as well as the intended process for manufacturing the drug.

The NDA has formed the basis for regulating and controlling new drugs in the United States since the passage of the Food, Drug, and Cosmetic Act (FD&C) in 1938. Since that time, various amendments to the FD&C have gradually increased the standards of evidence required to obtain approval.

One consequence of these more stringent standards is that the approval process can become very time consuming. The goal of the FDA's Center for Drug Evaluation and Research (CDER) is to review and act on at least 90% of NDAs for standard drugs within 10 months after the applications are received, and six months for priority drugs. Of course, the full timeline for drug development will frequently stretch to a decade or more.

Advantages and Disadvantages of the New Drug Application

The NDA submission process is just one phase of a multi-step process that pharmaceutical companies must navigate in order to successfully bring a new drug to market. From the perspective of the FDA, this rigorous process is necessary in order to protect the public from harmful or misleading drugs. On the other hand, many have argued that the new drug approval process is excessively onerous, posing a barrier to innovation and causing upward pressure on drug prices.

(447 words)

Reading A
Words and
Expressions

Words and Expressions			
commercialization	/kəˌmɜːʃəlaiˈzeiʃn/	n.	商品化，商业化
comprehensive	/ˌkɒmpriˈhensiv/	adj.	综合的；广泛的
vehicle	/ˈviːəkl/	n.	媒介；工具；车辆
sponsor	/ˈspɒnsə(r)/	n.	赞助商；主办者
		vt.	赞助；发起
propose	/prəˈpəʊz/	vt.	提出，计划
investigational	/inˌvestiˈgeiʃnəl/	adj.	试验性的
milestone	/ˈmailstəʊn/	n.	里程碑，划时代的事件
likelihood	/ˈlaiklihʊd/	n.	可能性，可能
evidence	/ˈevidəns/	n.	证据，证明
		vt.	证明
demonstrate	/ˈdemənstreit/	vt.	证明；展示；论证
manufacture	/ˌmænjuˈfæktʃə(r)/	n.	制造；产品；制造业
		vt.	制造；加工
amendment	/əˈmendmənt/	n.	修正案；改善；改正
stringent	/ˈstrindʒənt/	adj.	严格的；严厉的
evaluation	/iˌvæljuˈeiʃn/	n.	评价；评估
priority	/praiˈɒrəti/	n.	优先；优先权
stretch	/stretʃ/	v.	延长；伸展；延续
navigate	/ˈnævigeit/	vt.	进行；行驶；航行
perspective	/pəˈspektiv/	n.	观点；角度
rigorous	/ˈrigərəs/	adj.	严格的，严厉的；严酷的
misleading	/ˌmisˈliːdiŋ/	adj.	误导的；让人产生错误观念的

续表

onerous	/ˈəʊnərəs/	adj.	繁重的；麻烦的
barrier	/ˈbæriə(r)/	n.	障碍物，屏障；界线
innovation	/ˌɪnəˈveɪʃn/	n.	创新，革新；新方法
Proper Names			
New Drug Application（NDA）		新药申请	
the Food, Drug, and Cosmetic Act（FD&C）		《食品、药品和化妆品法》	
Center for Drug Evaluation and Research（CDER）		药物评估和研究中心	

📖 Notes

1. For decades, the regulation and control of new drugs in the United States has been based on the New Drug Application (NDA).

几十年来，美国对新药的监管和控制都是以新药申请为基础的。

"base on" 意为"基于，以……为根据；在……基础上"。

e. g. Your presentation should be based on the facts.

你的发言要以事实为根据。

2. A new drug application (NDA) is a comprehensive document that must be submitted to the U. S. Food and Drug Administration (FDA) in order to request approval for marketing a new drug in the United States.

新药申请是指为了申请批准在美国销售一种新药，向美国食品和药物管理局提交的一份综合文件。

"that" 作为关系代词引导定语从句，修饰先行词 "document"。

e. g. She is the girl that I saw last week.

她就是我上周见过的那个女孩。

3. It is the vehicle through which drug sponsors formally propose that the FDA approve a new pharmaceutical for sale and marketing in the U. S.

新药申请是药物赞助商正式提议美国食品和药物管理局批准一种新的药物在美国销售和营销的工具。

"through which" 介词加关系代词引导的定语从句，"through which" 即 "through the vehicle" 在从句中作状语。

e. g. Yesterday they visited the West Lake for which Hangzhou is famous.

昨天他们参观了以西湖而著名的杭州。

在定语从句中通常介词加关系代词相当于关系副词 where，when 或 why：

e. g. This is the village where (in which) he was born. 这就是他出生的村庄。

4. Yet, reaching the NDA stage is far from easy.

然而，达到新药申请这个阶段绝非易事。

"far from" 意为"远离"。

e. g. The airport is far from my office.

机场离我办公室很远。

5. One consequence of these more stringent standards is that the approval process can become very time consuming.

这些更严格的标准带来的一个后果就是审批过程变得非常耗时。

"that"引导表语从句。

e. g. The biggest headache problem was that he really misunderstood me.

最头疼的问题是他真的误解我了。

6. The NDA submission process is just one phase of a multi-step process that pharmaceutical companies must navigate in order to successfully bring a new drug to market.

制药公司必需要历经多个阶段才能成功的将一种新药推向市场，新药申请过程只是其中之一。

"multi-step"意为"多步骤的、多步的"，"multi""多种、多数"，可作为前缀。

e. g. multi-media 多媒体, multi-party 多党派, multi-staged 多层级。

7. From the perspective of the FDA, this rigorous process is necessary in order to protect the public from harmful or misleading drugs.

从美国食品和药物管理局的角度来看，为了保护公众免受药物损害或误导，这种严格的程序是必要的。

"protect…from…"意为"保护……免受……"

e. g. The body has natural defence mechanisms to protect it from disease.

人体对疾病有先天的防御机制。

After-reading Exercises

Task 1　Answer the following questions according to the text.

1. What is a New Drug Application?

_____

2. How many chapters does the NDA document must contain?

_____

3. What must be demonstrated in an NDA document?

_____

4. What are the goals of the FDA's Center for Drug Evaluation and Research for the approval process for priority drugs?

_____

5. What are the disadvantages of the New Drug Application?

_____

Task 2　Match the words（1-10）to the Chinese meanings（a-j）.

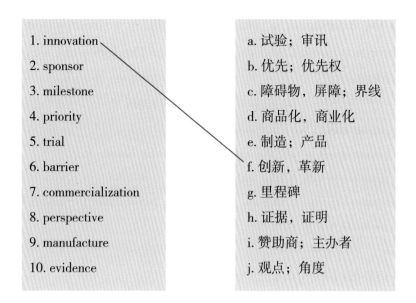

1. innovation
2. sponsor
3. milestone
4. priority
5. trial
6. barrier
7. commercialization
8. perspective
9. manufacture
10. evidence

a. 试验；审讯
b. 优先；优先权
c. 障碍物，屏障；界线
d. 商品化，商业化
e. 制造；产品
f. 创新，革新
g. 里程碑
h. 证据，证明
i. 赞助商；主办者
j. 观点；角度

Task 3　Fill in each blank with the proper form of the word or phrase given in brackets.

1. Nowadays, the _____ for studying is shifted from contents to methods.（priority）

2. The epidemic situation is difficult to _____ .（evaluation）

3. Last year, dozens of famous actors _____ the rescue event.（sponsor）

4. Bejing is a major center of cultural and _____ activity in China.（commercialization）

5. And most importantly, they have to learn how to _____ .（innovation）

Task 4　Translate the following sentences into English using the words or phrases you have learned in this unit.

1. 另一方面，许多人认为，新药审批流程过于繁琐，对创新构成障碍，对药品价格造成上行压力。（barrier）

_____

2. 几十年来，美国对新药的管理和控制都是以新药申请为基础的。（base on）

_____

3. 该文件必须广泛地证明所提议的药物的药理学、毒理学和剂量要求，以及制造药物的预期过程。（demonstrate）

_____

4. 然而，达到新药申请这个阶段绝非易事。（far from）

_____

5. 一旦提交了新药申请，这种药物通过美国食品和药物管理局批准的可能性通常会很高。（likelihood）

_____

Listening & Speaking

Task 1 At the drugstore, a pharmacist is filling a prescription for a patient. Listen to the conversation and decide whether the following statements are true（T）or false（F）.

Getting a Prescription Filled

(　) 1. The patient doesn't have a prescription.

(　) 2. The patient needs to take the medicine once a day before sleep.

(　) 3. The medicine is safe to take with aspirin.

(　) 4. If the patient forgets to take the pills the night before, take two tablets the next morning.

(　) 5. This medicine has no side effects.

📖 Notes

1. Please make up this prescription.

请按处方配药。

"make up a prescription" the same meaning as "fill a prescription", means the pharmacist dispense the medicine according to the doctor's prescription. （按照医生处方配药、抓药）。

e. g. The pharmacist is making up the prescription for patients.

药剂师正在给病人配药。

2. Are there any side effects?

有什么副作用吗?

"Side effect" refers to other pharmacological effects than for therapeutic purposes that occur after the application of a therapeutic dose of a drug.

在应用药物的治疗剂量后发生的除治疗目的以外的其他药理作用，即副作用。

e. g. The drug is known to have undesirable side effects.

众所周知，这种药有不良副作用。

3. It is recommended that you avoid physically demanding activities after taking this; also no driving.

建议在服药后避免体力活动；也不要开车。

" It is recommended that …" 引导的主语从句中要用虚拟语气，动词形式为 should ＋动词原形，should 可省略。

e. g. It is recommended that our schedule（should）be modified.

有人建议我们修改日程安排。

Task 2 At the drugstore, a pharmacist is receiving a patient without a doctor's prescription. Listen to the conversation and choose the best answer to each question you hear.

Buying Medicine without a Prescription

(　) 1. What's wrong with the patient?

　　　　A. Catch a cold　　　　　　　　B. Have a headache

C. Have a cough   D. All of the above

(　　) 2. What does the pharmacist suggest the patient drink?

A. Granule for treating cold   B. Radix isatidis granules

C. Hot tea with honey   D. None of the above

(　　) 3. Which of the following is a prescription drug?

A. Cough syrup   B. Penicillin

C. Pain killer   D. Throat lozenge

(　　) 4. Is the patient allergic to any type of medicine?

A. Yes, he is   B. No, he isn't

C. He doesn't know exactly   D. None of the above

(　　) 5. Decide the following statements, which one is correct?

A. The patient was diagnosed by the doctor as having a cold

B. The patient is allergic to penicillin

C. The patient does not need a doctor's prescription to buy penicillin

D. The patient needs to follow the instructions

📖 Notes

1. Are you allergic to any type of medication?

你对药物过敏吗?

be allergic to   对……过敏。

e. g. I'm allergic to milk and cheese.

我对牛奶和奶酪过敏。

2. penicillin   盘尼西林、青霉素。

3. cough syrup   止咳糖浆。

Task 3   The use of prescription is common in our life. Listen to the following passage and fill in the blanks with what you hear.

Make sure medication works safely to ＿＿＿＿1＿＿＿＿ your health, there are 8 drug DOs and DON'Ts for you to follow. DO take each medication ＿＿＿＿2＿＿＿＿ as it has been prescribed. DO make sure that all your doctors know about all your medications. DO keep medications out of the reach of children and pets. DON'T change your medication dose or ＿＿＿＿3＿＿＿＿ without talking with your doctor. DON'T use medication prescribed for someone else. DON'T crush or break pills unless your doctor ＿＿＿＿4＿＿＿＿ you to do so. DON'T use medication that has passed its ＿＿＿＿5＿＿＿＿ date. DON'T store your medications in locations that are humid, too hot or too cold.

Task 4   Work in groups, try to discuss the topic of "To buy drugs on / without a prescription". Practice making the conversations with your partner according to what you hear in the Listening part.

Listening &
Speaking
Task 3

医药大学堂
WWW.YIYAODXT.COM

Partner A	Partner B
Greet and reception.	Greet and requirements.
Confirm the prescription / symptoms.	Provide the prescription / complain about the symptoms.
Make up a prescription / recommend drugs.	Ask about the dosage.
Instruct the drug use.	Ask about the side effects.
Describe side effects and precautions.	Show the appreciation.

Reading B

Registration Routes of Imported Drugs in China

New drugs refer to drugs that have not been sold in or outside China. The imported drugs account for the vast majority of drugs approved for marketing in China. To market imported drugs, a developer must apply either for import drug license (IDL) ——the category III route, or conduct a full development program in China (the category I route) and submit a New Drug Application (NDA) for new drug approval.

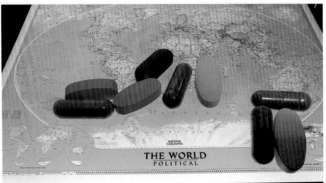

In choosing between these two routes, developers need to consider the importance of clinical trial application (CTA) review time, since an approved CTA is required for both. Of key importance is also the expected timeline of approval of the drug in the rest of the world as, by definition, a category I drug must not have been approved in any other country at time of NDA application. Therefore, The category III route (IDL) to registration is the most popular pathway to the Chinese market for pharmaceutical products.

The IDL requires a clinical trial conducted in Chinese subjects for registration of new chemical entities and for all new clinical indications. Normally, it is required that 100 pairs of subjects (i. e. 100 treated patients and 300 for biologics) are recruited in China for a clinical trial under the category Ⅲ IDL pathway, though this number can be subject to flexibility by the National Medical Produts Administration (NMPA). The number of pairs is dependent upon protocol, indication and trial design and must deliver the appropriate level of statistical significance to the study.

The NMPA's Provisions for Drug Registration permit the use of Chinese data from an international multicenter trial in the application for the IDL. More multinational developers are including Chinese trials in their global programs to gain access to large patient populations and collect data to support simultaneous registration in multiple countries, including China, using this IDL registration pathway. On average, developers conducting global multicenter development programs experience a four-to-six-year lag between the product's introduction in the U. S. and Europe and its introduction in China. This lag is due to the major differences in approval timelines, particularly for CTA reviews.

Given the limitations of the category Ⅲ IDL route, some developers are exploring the alternative——pursuing a category Ⅰ NDA based on a full development program in China. The category Ⅰ NDA is the default registration pathway for domestically-developed new drugs. The number of category Ⅰ NDA approvals is increasing, according to NMPA reports on annual drug registration. Category Ⅰ registration then requires Phase Ⅰ, Ⅱ and Ⅲ clinical trials to demonstrate safety and efficacy for the China NDA submission and NMPA review.

The first three steps in category Ⅰ registration take a minimum of two years to complete. CTA approval takes approximately one year, and NDA approval takes approximately two years. The total time frame is between four and five years. For registration via the category Ⅰ route using Chinese data from global multicenter trials, the timing could be less than 12 months after US/ EU approval, or, in some cases, could result in the first global approval.

China's hard-to-navigate drug approval system and slow processing have been major concerns of foreign biopharma companies. China is working on new measures that will shorten the time to market for approved imported drugs to speed up its drug approval process, according to the China Food and Drug Administration.

(563words)

Words and Expressions			
registration	/ˌredʒɪˈstreɪʃn/	n.	注册；登记；挂号
route	/ruːt/	n.	途径，渠道；路线
majority	/məˈdʒɒrəti/	n.	多数
license	/ˈlaɪsns/	n.	许可证，执照
conduct	/kənˈdʌkt/	v.	进行，组织，实施
entity	/ˈentəti/	n.	实体
recruit	/rɪˈkruːt/	v.	征募；聘用
flexibility	/ˌfleksəˈbɪləti/	n.	灵活性；弹性；适应性
deliver	/dɪˈlɪvə(r)/	vt.	提供；交付；递送
statistical	/stəˈtɪstɪkl/	adj.	统计的；统计学的

续表

simultaneous	/ˌsiml'teiniəs/	adj.	同时的；同时发生的
lag	/læg/	n.	落后；迟延
alternative	/ɔːl'tɜːnətiv/	adj.	供选择的；选择性的
		n.	二中择一；供选择的
default	/di'fɔːlt/	n.	默认；常规做法
domestically	/də'mestikli/	adv.	国内地
approximately	/ə'prɒksimətli/	adv.	大约，近于
biopharma	/ˌbaiəʊ'fɑːmə/	n.	生物制药

Proper Names

import drug license（IDL）	进口药品许可证
clinical trial application（CTA）	临床试验申请

After-reading Exercises

Task 1   Read the passage and choose the correct answer to each question.

(   ) 1. In China, there are _____ routes to register imported drugs.

     A. 1   B. 2

     C. 3   D. 4

(   ) 2. What kind of application for registration must be approved in China for imported drugs?

     A. Non-Disclosure Agreement

     B. New Drug Application

     C. Clinical Trial Application

     D. Investigational New Drug Application

(   ) 3. Why are more multinational developers including Chinese trials in their global programs?

     A. Gain access to large patient populations

     B. Collect more data

     C. Simultaneous registration in multiple countries

     D. All of the above

(   ) 4. The total timeframe of imported drugs applied for registration through the categoryⅢ IDL is generally _____ .

     A. 1-2 years   B. 2-3 years

     C. 3-4 years   D. 4-5 years

(   ) 5. According to the text, which of the following doesn't worry foreign biopharma companies?

     A. Drug approval funds   B. Drug approval system

     C. Drug approval process   D. Drug approval time

Task 2   Translate the following sentences into Chinese.

1. To market imported drugs, a developer must apply either for import drug license（IDL）——the category Ⅲ route, or conduct a full development program in China (the category Ⅰ route) and submit a

New Drug Application（NDA）for new drug approval.

2. The IDL requires a clinical trial conducted in Chinese subjects for registration of new chemical entities and for all new clinical indications.

3. The number of pairs is dependent upon protocol, indication and trial design and must deliver the appropriate level of statistical significance to the study.

4. More multinational developers are including Chinese trials in their global programs to gain access to large patient populations and collect data to support simultaneous registration in multiple countries, including China, using this IDL registration pathway.

5. China's hard-to-navigate drug approval system and slow processing have been major concerns of foreign biopharma companies.

Practical Writing

E-mail

电子邮件也叫电子函件，指通过互联网传递的邮件。一般由三部分构成，邮件头（E-mail header）、正文（Message content）和签名（Signature）。

Sample

From：sy347@cam.ac.uk

To：lna@sina.com

Cc：fxmary@online.sh.cn

Subject：New drugs recommended

Date：31st August, 2020

Attachments：new drug instruction

Dear Sir or Madam,

　　We are pleased to enclose a copy of our new drug instruction. Our new drug has just gone on sale after being approved by CFDA. It has better efficacy in clinical trials and a reasonable price. I believe you will have confidence in our drug.

　　We are looking forward to your orders.

Yours faithfully,

Zhou Shen

电子邮件通常包含以下内容：

邮件头：E-mail header；

寄件人的邮件地址：From；

收件人的邮件地址：To；

抄送（寄件人输入被抄送者邮件地址）：Cc（Carbon Copy）；

主题：Subject；

日期：Date；

附件：Attachments；

正文：Message content，邮件的内容，书写格式与常规信件相同；

签名：Signature，在邮件的最后一行。

Task Write an E-mail in English covering the following information.

1. 时间：2020 年 10 月 25 日；

2. 回复电子邮件样例；

3. 尝试订购新药；

4. 协商确定新药价格；

5. 期盼进一步合作。

From：_____

To：_____

Subject：_____

Date：_____

_____

_____

_____

_____

_____

_____

_____

Grammar Tips

状语从句（Adverbial Clause）是指句子用作状语时，起副词作用的句子。状语从句中的从句可以修饰谓语、非谓语动词，定语、状语或整个句子。状语从句根据其作用，可分为时间、地点、原因、条件、目的、结果、让步、方式和比较从句。状语从句一般由连词引导，也可由词组引起。从句位于句首和句中时通常用逗号与主句隔开，位于句尾时可不用逗号隔开。

Adverbial Clause

状语类别	从属连词
时间 Time	when, whenever, as, while, before, after, till, until, since, ever since, once, as soon as, soon after, the moment, the minutes, immediately, each time, last time, no sooner…than, hardly…when
	e. g. We have been friends since we met at the party.
地点 Place	where, wherever
	e. g. You'd better make a mark where you have any questions.
原因 Cause	because, as, since, considering, seeing that, now that
	e. g. Since you have no license, you are not allowed to drive.
目的 Purpose	so that, in order that, for fear that, in case, lest
	e. g. Take an umbrella in case it rains.
结果 Result	so that, so…that, such…that, with the result that
	e. g. What has happened that you look so anxious.
条件 Condition	if, unless, as long as, as far as, in case, suppose that, provided that, on condition that
	e. g. She won't be able to pass the exam unless she works hard.
比较 Comparison	as…as, not as…as, not so…as, than
	e. g. The result was not as good as I had expected.
让步 Concession	though, although, even if, even though, as, however, whatever, whenever, wherever, whoever, whether…or, no matter who/what/how/which/where/when/whether
	e. g. Though she was hungry, still she would not eat.
方式 Manner	as, as if, as though
	e. g. The boy plays piano as though he has s natural ear for music.

Task   Choose the best answer to complete each sentence according to the Adverbial Clause.

(   ) 1. ——Did Jack come back early last night?

    ——Yes. It was not yet eight o'clock _____ he arrived home.

    A. before   B. when

    C. that   D. until

(   ) 2. _____ I know the money is safe, I shall not worry about it.

    A. Even though   B. Unless

    C. As long as   D. While

(   ) 3. _____, his mother will wait for him to have dinner together.

    A. However late is he   B. However he is late

    C. However is he late   D. However late he is

(   ) 4. After the war, a new school building was put up _____ there had once been a theatre.

    A. that   B. where

    C. which   D. when

( ) 5. _____ you've got a chance, you might as well make full use of it.

    A. Now that   B. After

    C. Although   D. As soon as

( ) 6. I'd like to study law at university _____ my cousin prefers geography.

    A. though   B. as

    C. while   D. for

( ) 7. My parents live in a small village. They always keep candles in the house _____ there is a power cut.

    A. if   B. unless

    C. in case   D. so that

( ) 8. "You can't have this football back _____ you promise not to kick it at my cat again." the old man said firmly.

    A. because   B. since

    C. when   D. until

( ) 9. ——Did you remember to give Mary the money you owed her?

    ——Yes. I gave it to her _____ I saw her.

    A. while   B. the moment

    C. suddenly   D. once

( ) 10. He was about halfway through his meal _____ a familiar voice came to his ears.

    A. why   B. where

    C. when   D. while

( ) 11. ——Dad, I've finished my assignment.

    ——Good, and _____ you play or watch TV, you mustn't disturb me.

    A. whenever   B. whether

    C. whatever   D. no matter

( ) 12. You will be successful in the interview _____ you have confidence.

    A. before   B. once

    C. until   D. through

( ) 13. Many of then turned a deaf ear to his advice, _____ they knew it to be valuable.

    A. as if   B. now that

    C. even though   D. so that

( ) 14. _____, his idea was accepted by all the people at the meeting.

    A. Strange as might it sound   B. As it might sound strange

    C. As strange it might sound   D. Strange as it might sound

( ) 15. Generally speaking, _____ according to the directions, the drug has no side effects.

    A. when taking   B. when taken

    C. when to take   D. when to be taken

Supplementary Reading

Investigational New Drug in America

James Chen

May 1, 2018

In America, the term Investigational New Drug (IND) refers to a drug developed by a pharmaceutical or biotech company or other organization that is ready for clinical trials on humans.

Investigational New Drugs (INDs) fall into two categories——commercial and research INDs. The big difference between these two categories is who does the application filing. As the name suggests, the commercial IND category is sought by a company that wants to test a drug in order to bring it to market. Any company can apply for this IND. The research or non-commercial IND is the step investigators require to run tests on an existing drug. Researchers require approval when they want to test approved drugs that are already on the market. Testing may include new dosages or new applications for these drugs.

When a company develops a new drug, it must get approval from the FDA before it can sell it to the general public. The company must go through a series of steps and applications before it can get to this point. It's up to the company——which is also called the drug sponsor——to run the required tests, gather data, and to make sure patients aren't exposed to unnecessary risks when they take the drug. The FDA reviews the results after each phase and makes a determination of whether the drug is safe for the public.

And the most important part is clinical trials for Investigational Drugs. If the FDA gives the green light of the IND application, the investigational drug will then enter three phases of clinical trials:

Phase 1: About 20 to 80 healthy volunteers to establish a drug's safety and profile, and takes about 1 year. Safety, metabolism and excretion of the drug are also emphasized.

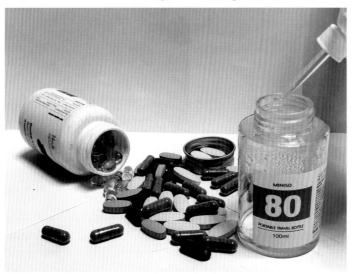

Phase 2: Roughly 100 to 300 patient volunteers to assess the drug's effectiveness in those with a specific condition or disease. This phase runs about 2 years. Groups of similar patients may receive the actual drug compared to a placebo (inactive pill) or other active drug to determine if the drug has an effect. Safety and side effects are reviewed.

Phase 3: Typically, several thousand patients are monitored in clinics and hospitals to carefully determine effectiveness and identify further side effects. Different types and age ranges of patients are evaluated. The manufacturer may look at different doses as well as the experimental drug in combination with other treatments. This phase runs about 3 years on average.

The clinical trials can cost hundreds of millions of dollars——and many years——to undertake clinical trials to bring a new drugto market. The IND application signifies that the sponsor is willing to make this huge investment. As such, investor reaction to an IND application——which is merely the first step in a long and arduous process for drug approval——is typically neutral.

(James Chen is the director of Trading & Investing Content at Investopedia.)

(472 words)

After-reading Exercises

Task Decide whether the following statements are true (T) or false (F) according to the text.

( ) 1. In the United States, there are two types of Investigational New Drugs (INDs): commercial INDs and research INDs.

( ) 2. The commercial IND is the step investigators require to run tests on an existing drug.

( ) 3. If the FDA gives the green light of the IND application, the investigational drug will then enter two phases of clinical trials.

( ) 4. The first phase needs about 20 to 80 healthy volunteers to establish a drug's safety and profile, it takes about 1 year.

( ) 5. The investors' reaction to an IND application is typically neutral.

Vocabulary Tips

Root "-naut-, -nav-": 船。-naut-来源于希腊语 naus（船）；-nav-来源于拉丁语中 navis（船）。

Example: navy 海军；navigate 驾驶，航海；nausea 作呕，晕船；astronavigation 宇宙航行。

Root "bio-, bi-": 生命，生物。

Example: biopharma 生物制药；biochemistry 生物化学；biocide 杀虫剂；microbe 细菌，微生物（micro 微小 + be = bi 生命）；autobiography 自传。

Task Complete the sentences with the given words.

navigate	autobiography	biochemistry	nausea	biocide

1. She feels _____ and aches in her muscles.

2. Study shows that the effectiveness of a compound _____ is better, and the dosage used to be small.

3. You know _____ goes far beyond oxygen.

4. The river became too narrow and shallow to _____.

5. Her new book is a continuation of her _____.

Proverbs and Sayings

◇An ounce of prevention is worth a pound of cure.

　一份预防方，胜过百份药。

◇Three points to take medicine, seven points conditioning.

　三分吃药，七分调理。

◇There is no great or low prescription, but the effective is a panacea.

　药方无贵贱，效者是灵丹。

题库

Unit **7**

Drug Safety

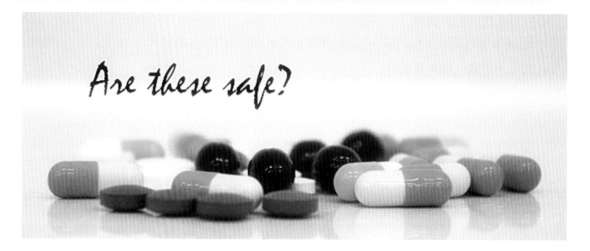

Are these safe?

Unit Objectives

After studying this unit, you are expected to:

· master the vocabulary and technical terms related to drug safety;

· understand the importance of drug safety and the health hazards may caused by drug abuse;

· know English tenses correctly.

And you should learn how to:

· communicate with others about prevention of drug adverse events and making instruction in drug use;

· write a medication package insert.

Introduction

Drug safety (also known as pharmacovigilance), is the science of detection, assessment, understanding and prevention of side effects which allows us to understand more about the risks and benefits of a medicine.

Pharmacovigilance heavily focuses on adverse drug reactions, or ADRs, which are defined as any response to a drug which is noxious and unintended, including lack of efficacy (the condition that this definition only applies with the doses normally used for the prophylaxis, diagnosis or therapy of disease, or for the modification of physiological disorder function was excluded with the latest amendment of the applicable legislation). Medication errors such as overdose, and misuse and abuse of a drug as well as drug exposure during pregnancy and breastfeeding, are also of interest, even without an adverse event, because they may result in an adverse drug reaction.

Warming-up

Task Work in groups. Look at the medications labels and match them to the proper meanings. Then check your answers with your partner.

FOR EXTERNAL USE
ONLY

A

SHAKE WELL
BEFORE USING

B

DO NOT DRINK
ALCOHOLIC BEVERAGES
WHEN TAKING THIS MEDICATION

C

KEEP in REFRIGERATOR
DO NOT FREEZE

D

(   ) 1. With some medications, even one drink can pose hazards. You may need to abstain from alcohol before or after taking these drugs.

(   ) 2. The medicine is intended to be used only on the outside of your body, and not to be eaten or drunk.

(   ) 3. The medicine is sensitive to high temperature and must be stored in the refrigerator, normally at 2-8℃.

(   ) 4. It is generally used for a liquid-liquid solution which is a non-homogeneous mixture. Move the solution up and down or back and forth with short quick movements before taking it.

Reading A

Overuse Makes Antibiotics Anti-health

Reading A

Imagine you have bacterial infection and all the antibiotics prescribed by doctors in the hospital cannot cure it. This is no science fiction scenario about "superbugs"; it is actually happening worldwide. Improper or overuse of antibiotics is proven to be the leading cause of public health problems.

Overuse of Antibiotics in China

China accounts for half of the antibiotics consumed worldwide, half for humans and the rest for food animals. Antibiotics for long have been available in the country's hospitals to prevent post-surgery and other infections. They are also available over the counter at drug stores which people use for self-treatment-for conditions like cough or a running nose.

医药大学堂
WWW.YIYAODXT.COM

Public health experts say the more antibiotics a person has taken the greater the risk he/she has to be infected by superbugs, and urge for strengthened and coordinated government efforts to stop the misuse and address the challenge.

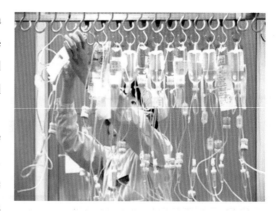

The Review on Anti-microbial Resistance (AMR), published in the United Kingdom this year, estimates that by 2050, AMR (including antibiotic resistance) could cause 1 million premature deaths a year in China.

Coordinated Action to AMR prevention in China

China's decision-makers have recognized the looming crisis and decided to take coordinated action to prevent it. A state-level action plan on AMR prevention and control will be issued by more than 10 departments, including the National Health and Family Planning Commission, China Food and Drug Administration, and Ministry of Education of the People's Republic of China.

Xiao Yonghong, a professor at the Institute of Clinical Pharmacology at Peking University, says the long overdue initiative shows the government's determination to tackle the issue head on.

Previously, the health authorities largely initiated the measures to fight AMR, which included stricter control of antibiotic usage at medical facilities. For instance, East China's Jiangsu province became the first province to issue a blanket ban on the use of intravenous antibiotics on outpatients at 2015. And provincial health authorities say the ban is working with public awareness about overuse of antibiotics increasing. Other provinces like Zhejiang, Jiangxi and Anhui are likely to follow suit soon. But that's far from enough.

The misuse of antibiotics in the agricultural sector is still widespread, which has been noted by many Chinese experts and even in the UK report on AMR.

To prevent infections in and boost the growth of food animals——most of them reared on feces-filled, cramped farms——operators regularly feed them antibiotics. This has turned the farms into fertile breeding grounds for drug-resistant pathogens that could also threaten humans.

Remember a joint China-US study in 2013? It found "diverse and abundant antibiotic-resistant genes in Chinese pig farms", which could contaminate the soil and water and migrate to humans through food. So, the fight against AMR cannot be won without the active involvement of the agriculture sector, for which the use of antibiotics in food animals must be drastically curbed.

Other stakeholders like the environment and education authorities, too, have to join the fight by monitoring the antibiotics contamination level and helping raise public awareness.

Global War on AMR Need China

There's still a long way to go and the expected government action plan would be a good start to the all-out war on AMR in China. That will also help China fulfill its international responsibility in public health. China has to be part of the global fight against AMR. And the global war on AMR cannot be won without China.

(553 words)

Words and Expressions

overuse	/ˌəʊvəˈjuːz/	n.	过度使用
antibiotic	/ˌæntibaiˈɒtik/	n.	抗生素
bacterial	/bækˈtiəriəl/	adj.	细菌的
infection	/inˈfekʃən/	n.	感染
prescribe	/priˈskraib/	vt.	开处方
superbug	/ˈsuːpəbʌɡ/	n.	超级细菌
self-treatment	/self ˈtriːtmənt/	n.	自我治疗
condition	/kənˈdiʃən/	n.	情况
misuse	/ˌmisˈjuːz/	n.	误用；滥用
premature	/ˈpremətʃər/	n.	早产儿
looming	/ˈluːmiŋ/	adj.	（不希望的事情）逼近的
state-level	/steit ˈlevl/	adj.	国家级
overdue	/ˌəʊvəˈdʒuː/	adj.	早该发生的
initiative	/iˈniʃətiv/	n.	（重要的）法案；倡议
tackle	/ˈtækl /	vt.	处理（难题或局面）
authority	/ɔːˈθɒrəti/	n.	权威；当局
facility	/fəˈsiləti/	n.	机构
blanket	/ˈblæŋkit/	adj.	没有限制的
ban	/bæn/	n.	禁令
outpatient	/ˈaʊtpeiʃnt/	n.	门诊病人
awareness	/əˈweənəs/	n.	意识
widespread	/ˈwaidspred/	adj.	普遍的；广泛的
rear	/riə (r) /	vt.	喂养；培养
cramped	/ kræmpt/	adj.	狭窄的
fertile	/ˈfɜːtail/	adj.	能生育的
diverse	/daiˈvɜːs/	adj.	多种多样的
contaminate	/kənˈtæmineit/	n.	污染
migrate	/maiˈɡreit/	vt.	迁徙；移动
curb	/kɜːb/	vt.	控制；抑制
stakeholder	/ˈsteikhəʊldə(r) /	n.	利益相关者

Proper Names

Anti-microbial Resistance（AMR）	抗微生物药物耐药性
the National Health and Family Planning Commission	国家卫生和计划生育委员会
Peking University	北京大学

📖 Notes

1. …the more antibiotics a person has taken the greater the risk he/she has to be infected by superbugs.

抗生素使用量越多，人类被超级细菌感染的风险就越大。

"the more… the more…"句型为"the + 比较级，the + 比较级"，通常表示"越……越……"，是一个复合句，前面的句子是状语从句，后面的句子是主句。The 用在形容词或副词的比较级前。

e. g. The harder you work, the greater progress you will make.

你越用功，进步就越大。

2. The Review on Anti-microbial Resistance（AMR），published in the United Kingdom this year, estimates that by 2050, AMR（including antibiotic resistance）could cause 1 million premature deaths a year in China.

今年在英国出版的《抗微生物药物耐药性评论》（AMR）估计：到 2050 年，中国每年将有 100 万人由于 AMR（包括抗生素抗药性）而早逝。

"published in the United Kingdom this year"省略了"which is"，是一个非限制性定语从句，修饰主语"the review"。非限制性定语从句与先行词关系不十分密切，只是对其作一些附加说明，不起限定制约的作用，如果将非限制性定语从句省去，主句的意义仍然完整。

e. g. Mr. Zhang, who came to see me yesterday, is an old friend of mine.

昨天来看我的张先生，他是我的一位老朋友。

"premature death"英文解释为"deaths that occurs before the average age of death in a certain population"意为"在某一特定人群中，死亡年龄低于平均死亡年龄"即为"过早死亡；早逝"。

e. g. Scoot pollution can irritate the lungs, worsen conditions like asthma and increase the risks of heart attacks and premature death.

煤烟污染会刺激肺部，加重哮喘等疾病，增加心脏病发作和过早死亡的风险。

3. To prevent infections in and boost the growth of food animals——most of them reared on feces-filled, cramped farms——operators regularly feed them antibiotics.

为防止食用动物感染疾病并促进它们的生长（大部分食用动物都饲养在满是粪便，拥挤不堪的农场中），农场主定期给它们喂服抗生素。

"——most of them reared on feces-filled, cramped farms——"，该句子的成分为插入语，一般破折号用在一个解释性的插入语的前面和后面（相当于一个括号）。

e. g. During my vacation——I must have been insane——I decided I would ski.

假期中，我准是疯了，决定去滑雪。

4. It found "diverse and abundant antibiotic-resistant genes in Chinese pig farms", which could contaminate the soil and water and migrate to humans through food.

它发现了"中国养猪场中存在大量多样的耐药基因"，这些基因可能污染土壤和水，并通过食物迁移到人类。

"antibiotic-resistant genes"意为"耐药基因"，是一种病毒基因，携带基因的病菌免疫部分抗生素，有耐药性。

e. g. The distribution, characterization and effect on antibiotic resistant gene dissemination of the integron among 59 Cefoxitin-resistance Escherichia coli clinical isolated strains were investigated.

研究临床分离的 59 株耐头孢西汀大肠埃希菌整合子的结构、分布及其在耐药基因播散中的作用。

After-reading Exercises

Task 1　Answer the following questions according to the text.

1. How have antibiotics been used in China for long time?

_____

2. According to public health experts' opinions, what will happen if a person takes a great amount of antibiotics?

_____

3. Why does agricultural sector play an important role in combatting AMR?

_____

4. Can you give some examples of the measures environment and education can take to fight against AMR?

_____

5. What does "AMR" refer to according to the passage?

_____

Task 2　Match the words (1-10) to the Chinese meanings (a-j).

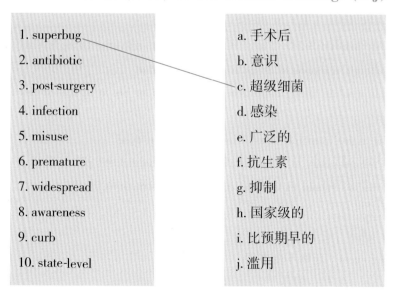

1. superbug
2. antibiotic
3. post-surgery
4. infection
5. misuse
6. premature
7. widespread
8. awareness
9. curb
10. state-level

a. 手术后
b. 意识
c. 超级细菌
d. 感染
e. 广泛的
f. 抗生素
g. 抑制
h. 国家级的
i. 比预期早的
j. 滥用

Task 3　Fill in each blank with the proper form of the word or phrase given in brackets.

1. It was found harmful and even life-threatening of _____ prescription drugs. (misuse)
2. Last year smoking in all public places was _____ . (ban)
3. A single mosquito can _____ a large number of people. (infection)
4. To assess the drivers of viral _____ , we run a variety of tests. (migrate)

医药大学堂
WWW.YIYAODXT.COM

5. Danny was born _____, weighing only 3lb 3oz.（premature）

Task 4   Translate the following sentences into English using the words or phrases you have learned in this unit.

1. 抗生素使用不当或过度使用是造成公共卫生问题的主要原因。（overuse）

_____

2. 想象一下有一天，你被细菌感染而医生开的所有抗生素都无法治愈。（prescribe）

_____

3. 人们也可以到药店直接买到抗生素用于自我治疗，比如治疗咳嗽或者流鼻涕。（self treatment）

_____

4. 这些耐药基因可能污染土壤和水。（contaminate）

_____

5. 环境和教育部门可通过监测抗生素污染水平及提高公众意识，参与到这场斗争中。（public awareness）

_____

Listening & Speaking

Listening &
Speaking
Task 1

Task 1   A pharmacology instructor is teaching a student about medication safety. Listen to the conversation and decide whether the following statements are true（T）or false（F）.

Medication Safety Tips：How to Prevent Adverse Drug Events？

（   ）1. All allergic reactions to drugs are not preventable.

（   ）2. People who are taking more than four medications are at increased risk for an adverse drug event.

（   ）3. 'Five rights' principle doesn't include the right dose.

（   ）4. It is not necessary to write the allergies and pharmacist's phone number on the list.

（   ）5. Pharmacists should make detailed drug use instructions for the patients.

📖 **Notes**

1. medication safety   安全用药。

2. adverse drug event   药物不良事件。

3. dispense drugs   发药；摆药。

4. 'five rights' principle   安全用药的"五个准确"，包括准确的病人，准确的药物，准确的剂量，准确的给药途径和准确的给药时间。

Listening &
Speaking
Task 2

Task 2   A pharmacist is instructing a patient's mother about how to take drugs correctly. Listen to the conversation and choose the best answer to each question you hear.

Making an Instruction in Drug Use

(　) 1. Why does the pharmacist recommend storing the drug in the fridge?

　　A. The drug will taste good in the fridge

　　B. The drug will go bad if you put it at room temperature

　　C. The drug can extend storage time in the fridge

　　D. Not mentioned

(　) 2. Which step is not correct when the mother feeds her baby with the drug?

　　A. She should prepare a spoon or a syringe

　　B. She should stop the medication when her baby feels better

　　C. She should put the seven mils medication in two to three times

　　D. She should vibrate the medication bottle thoroughly to mix the ingredients

(　) 3. How long will the full course last?

　　A. 7 days　　　　　　　B. 12 hours

　　C. 10 hours　　　　　　D. 10 days

(　) 4. Which is not the reason for the full course therapy?

　　A. stop the relapse of the infection

　　B. reduce the risk of the bacterial becoming resistant to the antibiotics

　　C. reduce the risk of the side effects

　　D. make sure the infection clears up

(　) 5. Decide the following statements, which one is correct?

　　A. The drug is amoxicillin to eradicate the ear infection

　　B. It will not cause aspiration even the daughter takes all the seven mils at once

　　C. The mom will not follow the order of the pharmacist

　　D. The doctor had already explained everything about the drug to the mom

📖 **Notes**

1. Amoxicillin　阿莫西林，青霉素类抗生素。

2. The full course therapy will stop the infection from returning, as well as reduce the risk of the bacterial becoming resistant to the antibiotics.

完成整个疗程的治疗不但能降低细菌对抗生素产生耐药性的危险，还可以防止感染的复发。

"as well as"：也；不但…而且。

e. g. The boy has learned to speak English as well as read some English books.

这个男孩不仅读了一些英语书而且学会了说英语。

Task 3　Drug safety is one of the hottest topics in daily medical practice. Listen to the following passage and fill in the blanks with what you hear.

In the U. S. , the government's Food and Drug Administration (FDA) must approve any drug before it can be sold. This is true whether it's a ____1____ or an ____2____ drug. The FDA evaluates the safety of a drug by looking at side effects: how it's ____3____ and results of animal testing and clinical ____4____ The FDA also ____5____ a drug's safety after approval. For you,

Listening &

Speaking

Task 3

drug safety means buying online from only legitimate pharmacies and taking your medicines correctly.

Task 4 **Work in groups, try to discuss the topic of "How to prevent adverse drug events?" and "Make an instruction in drug use." Practice making the conversations with your partner according to what you hear in the listening part.**

Partner A	Partner B
Greet.	Greet and ask the adverse drug event.
Introduce the adverse drug event.	Ask who are at risk for adverse drug events.
Answer the question correctly.	Ask how to prevent adverse drug events.
Tell the ways to prevent adverse drug events.	An instruction in drug use.
Explain the detailed information of drug to the patients.	Show the understanding and appreciation.

Reading B

The Package Insert of Tylenol

TYLENOL EXTRA STRENGTH—acetaminophen tablet, film coated

Navajo Manufacturing Company Inc.

Name

Generic Name : Acetaminophen

Brand Name : Tylenol

Active Ingredients (in each caplet)

Acetaminophen 500 mg

Purpose

Pain reliever/fever reducer

Uses

· temporarily relieves minor aches and pains due to:

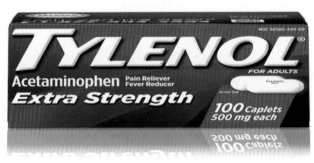

- the common cold   · headache   · backache
- minor pain of arthritis   · toothache   · muscular aches
- premenstrual and menstrual cramps
- temporarily reduces fevers

Warnings

Liver warning: This product contains acetaminophen. Severe liver damage may occur if you take
- more than 4,000 mg of acetaminophen in 24 hours
- with other drugs containing acetaminophen
- 3 or more alcoholic drinks every day while using this product

Allergy alert: acetaminophen may cause severe skin reactions. Symptoms may include:
- skin reddening · blisters · rash

If a skin reaction occurs, stop use and seek medical help right away.

Do not use
- with any other drug containing acetaminophen (prescription or nonprescription). If you are not sure whether a drug contains acetaminophen, ask a doctor or pharmacist.
- if you are allergic to acetaminophen or any of the inactive ingredients in this product

Ask a doctor before use if you have liver disease.

Ask a doctor or pharmacist before use if you are taking the blood thinning drug warfarin.

Stop use and ask a doctor if
- pain gets worse or lasts more than 10 days
- fever gets worse or lasts more than 3 days
- new symptoms occur
- redness or swelling is present

These could be signs of a serious condition.

If pregnant or breast-feeding, ask a health professional before use.

Keep out of reach of children.

Overdose warning: In case of overdose, get medical help or contact a Poison Control Center right away. (1-800-222-1222) Quick medical attention is critical for adults as well as for children even if you do not notice any signs or symptoms.

Directions

· Do not take more than directed (see overdose warning)

adults and children 12 years and over	· take 2 caplets every 6 hours while symptoms last · do not take more than 6 caplets in 24 hours, unless directed by a doctor · do not use for more than 10 days unless directed by a doctor
children under 12 years	· ask a doctor

Other information

· store between 20-25°C（68-77°F）

· see bottom of carton for lot number and expiration date

· do not use if pouch is opened

Inactive ingredients

carnauba wax＊, corn starch, FD&C red no. 40 aluminum lake, hypromellose, magnesium stearate, polyethylene glycol＊, powdered cellulose, pregelatinized starch, propylene glycol, shellac, sodium starch glycolate, titanium dioxide

＊contains one or more of these ingredients

Questions or comments?

call 1-877-895-3665（toll-free）or 215-273-8755（collect）

（428 words）

Words and Expressions			
ingredient	/in'griːdiənt/	n.	原料；要素；组成部分
caplet	/'kæplət/	n.	囊片
minor	/'mainər/	adj.	次要的；轻微的
ache	/eik/	n.	（身体某部位）疼痛
pain	/pein /	n.	疼痛
arthritis	/ɑː'θraitis/	n.	关节炎
premenstrual	/priː'menstruəl/	adj.	月经前的；经期前的
cramp	/kræmp/	n.	痉挛；绞痛
liver	/'livər/	n.	肝脏
alcoholic	/ælkə'hɒlik/	adj.	酒精的；含酒精的
redden	/'redn/	v.	（使）变红
blister	/'blistər/	n.	水疱
rash	/ræʃ/	n.	（皮肤）皮疹
swelling	/'sweliŋ/	n.	肿胀
pregnant	/'pregnənt/	adj.	怀孕的
breast-feeding	/brest 'fiːdiŋ/	vt.	用母乳喂养
overdose	/'əʊvədəʊs/	n.	药量过多

Proper Names	
Tylenol	泰诺
Generic Name	通用名
Acetaminophen	对乙酰氨基酚
Brand Name	商品名
warfarin	华法林（一种抗凝血剂）
Poison Control Center	中毒控制中心
Lot number	批号

After-reading Exercises

Task 1　Read the passage and choose the correct answer to each question.

(　)　1.　The purposes of Tylenol are not include _____ .

      A.　relieving headache　　　　　　B.　reducing fever

      C.　relieving premenstrual cramps　　D.　treating an infection

(　)　2.　If severe skin reactions occur, you may have the following symptoms except _____ .

      A.　skin reddening　　　　　　　　B.　blisters

      C.　rash　　　　　　　　　　　　　D.　skin dryness

(　)　3.　According to the passage, you should stop using the drug if _____ .

      A.　pain lasts more than 3 days

      B.　new symptoms occur

      C.　fever lasts more than 1 days

      D.　pale is present

(　)　4.　For the patients who are children 12 years and over, which drug direction is correct?

      A.　You must ask a doctor

      B.　You can take the drug as long as you want

      C.　Take 2 caplets every 6 hours as far as you are still feverish

      D.　If you have a high fever, you should take 2 caplets every 6 hours until you feel better

(　)　5.　Which statement is wrong according to the passage?

      A.　The drugcan be stored at 23℃

      B.　Do not use the drug if you have liver disease

      C.　Do not use if the package is opened

      D.　Consult with a doctor if you are taking warfarin

Task 2　Translate the following sentences into Chinese.

1.　Severe liver damage may occur if you take more than 4,000 mg of acetaminophen in 24 hours.

_____

2.　It can temporarily relieve minor aches and pains due to arthritis.

_____

3.　Acetaminophen may cause severe skin reactions which may include skin reddening, blister, and rash.

_____

4.　Ask a doctor or pharmacist before use if you are taking the blood thinning drug warfarin.

_____

5.　In case of overdose, get medical help or contact a Poison Control Center right away.

_____

Practical Writing

A Drug Package Insert

药品说明书是载明药品的重要信息的法定文件，是选用药品的法定指南。新药审批后的说明书，不得自行修改。药品说明书的内容应包括药品的品名、规格、生产企业、药品批准文号、产品批号、有效期、主要成分、适应证或功能主治、用法、用量、禁忌、不良反应和注意事项，中药制剂说明书还应包括主要药味（成分）性状、药理作用、贮藏等。

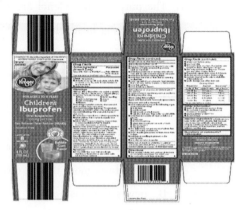

Sample

LianHua QingWen Capsule

Generic Name：Lianhua Qingwen Jiaonang

Trade Name：Yiling

Ingredients：Weeping Forsythia Capsule, Japanese Honeysuckle Flower, Ephedra Herb（honey-fried）, Bitter Apricot Seed（stir-baked）, Gypsum, Isatis Root, Male Fern Rhizome, Heartleaf Houttuynia Herb, Cablin Patchouli Herb, Rhubarb, Bigflower Rhodiola Root, Menthol, Liquorice Root.

Functions and Indications：Clear heat and detoxify, remove lung hotness. Used in treatment of epidemic influenza and lung heat, symptom as fever or high fever, aversion to cold, muscular soreness, rhinostegnosis and nasal discharge, or yellow or greasy fur of tongue.

Description：Capsules, containing tan to brown granules and powders; odor, slightly aromatic; taste slightly bitter.

Strength：0.35g/Capsule.

Administration and Dosage：For oral administration, 4 capsules once, 3 times daily.

Adverse Reactions：Uncertain.

Contraindications：Uncertain.

Note：

1. Avoid smoking, alcohol and spicy, cold and greasy food.

2. It is not suitable to take tonic Chinese medicine at the same time.

3. Not suitable for people with cold.

4. Patients with hypertension and heart disease should use it with caution. Those with serious chronic diseases such as liver disease, diabetes mellitus and kidney disease should take it under the guidance of doctors.

5. Children, pregnant women, breast-feeding women, old and weak, and those with spleen deficiency and loose stools should be taken under the guidance of doctors.

6. Patients with fever temperature over 38.5℃ should go to the hospital for treatment.

7. Take it in strict accordance with the usage and dosage. This product is not suitable for long-term use.

8. If the symptoms are not relieved after taking the medicine for 3 days, you should go to the hospital.

9. It is forbidden to use this product in case of allergy, and it should be used with caution in case of allergic constitution.

10. It is forbidden to use this product when its properties change.

11. Children must be used under adult supervision.

12. Please keep this product out of the reach of children.

13. If you are using other drugs, please consult a doctor or pharmacist before using this product.

14. Athletes should be careful.

15. After opening the moisture-proof bag, please pay attention to moisture proof.

Package：Aluminum-plastic blister package.

Storage：Preserve in tightly closed containers, stored in a cool and dry place（≤20℃）.

Shelf life：30 Months（Expiry Date：≥24 Months）.

药品说明书通常包含以下项目：

通用名：Generic Name；

商品名：Trade Name；

药物成分：Ingredients；

功能和适应证：Functions and Indications；

性状：Description；

规格：Strength；

用法用量：Administration and Dosage；

副作用：Adverse Reactions；

禁忌证：Contraindications；

注意事项：Note；

包装：Package；

储存：Storage；

保质期：Shelf life。

Task　A pharmacology instructor has taught some basic information about Rosuvastatin Calcium Tablets. Please try to write a drug package insert of Rosuvastatin Calcium Tablets according to the information given below in Chinese.

瑞舒伐他汀钙片，商品名为可定，成分的分子式是（$C_{22}H_{27}FN_3O_6S$）$_2$Ca，粉红色薄膜衣片。适用于高三酰甘油血症（Hypertriglyceridemia）、原发性血脂异常蛋白血症（Primary Dysbetalipoproteinemia）和纯合子家族性高胆固醇血症（Homozygous Familial Hypercholesterolemia）。产品规格为5mg/片，共7片。常见的不良反应包括头痛、无力、肌痛、恶心和腹痛。服用方法为口服，一次服用剂量时5mg，一日一次。本品禁用于对瑞舒伐他汀成分过敏者、活动性肝病患者、严重的肾功能损坏的患者、妊娠期和哺乳期女性。如果出现皮肤发黄或者呼吸短促，不明原因的咳嗽，以及全身无力，请立即去医院。本品为铝/铝塑泡包装，有效期36个月，密封，在干燥处保存。

Rosuvastatin Calcium

Generic Name：_____

Trade Name：_____

Ingredients：_____

Functions and Indications：_____

Description：_____

Strength：_____

Administration and Dosage：_____

Adverse Reactions：_____

Contraindications：_____

Note：_____

Package：_____

Storage：_____

Shelf life：_____

Grammar Tips

　　时态（tense）是一种动词形式，不同的时态用以表示不同的时间与方式。它是表示行为、动作、状态在各种时间条件下的动词形式。

Tenses

时态	定义	构成
一般现在时 Simple Present Tense	无时限或现在的动作或状态	动词原形；主语是第三人称单数，用动词的第三人称单数形式
	e. g. He feels tired all the time.	
一般过去时 Simple Past Tense	表示过去的动作或状态	过去式
	e. g. She presented to her GP with chest pain.	
一般将来时 Simple Future Tense	表示将要发生的动作或状态	1. will（shall）＋动词原形 2. am/is/are ＋ going ＋ to＋动词原形 3. am/is/are＋不定式 4. am/is/are ＋ about＋动词不定式 5. 现在进行时，一般现在时表一般将来时
	e. g. He will make a full recovery soon.	
过去将来时 Past Future Tense	表示过去时间内将要发生的事情	1. would（should）＋动词原形 2. was/were＋ going ＋ to＋动词原形
	e. g. She and I were to meet at an agreed place.	
现在进行时 Present Continuous Tense	现在正在进行的动作	am/is/are ＋现在分词
	e. g. I'm having difficulty swallowing solid food.	

续表

时态	定义	构成
过去进行时 Past Continuous Tense	表示过去正在进行的动作	was/were + 现在分词
	e. g. She broke her leg when she was leaving the office.	
将来进行时 Future Continuous Tense	将来某一时间正在进行的动作	will（shall）be + 现在分词
	e. g. This time next day they will be sitting in the cinema.	
现在完成时 Present Perfect Tense	1. 动作发生在过去，对现在有影响 2. 动作发生在过去，一直持续到现在	have/has + 现在分词
	e. g. She has had lots of plastic surgery.	
过去完成时 Past Perfect Tense	过去某一时间或动作以前已经发生了或完成了的动作	had + 过去分词
	e. g. He had an operation for colon cancer last summer.	
将来完成时 Future Perfect Tense	到将来某个时刻为止已经完成的动作	will（shall）have + 过去分词
	e. g. By the end of the month, he will have been living here for ten years.	
现在完成进行时 Present Perfect Progressive Tense	强调从过去到现在一直在进行的动作	have/has been + 现在分词
	e. g. It has been raining for two days.	
过去完成进行时 Past Perfect Progressive Tense	过去的过去在一直进行的动作	had been + 现在分词
	e. g. He had been suffering from a bad cold when she took the exam.	

Task 1   Complete the sentences with the correct grammatical form of verb.

1. Biopsy of the pancreas _____ last March. （perform）

2. A number of studies _____ recently to look at this question. （carry out）

3. The patient usually _____ with a severe sore throat. （present）

4. She _____ 9 kg in weight last year before she came to the hospital. （gain）

5. The doctor asked what he _____. （eat）

6. They _____ for 20 years by then. （marry）

7. Stop the patient or he _____. （fall over）

8. The doctor _____ the bowel sound now. （listen）

9. Last Sunday we _____ the Great Wall, but it rained. （visit）

10. In this case, the patient _____ that he had not been taking the drugs regularly. （admit）

Task 2   Choose the best answer to complete each sentence according to the Tenses.

(   ) 1. The teacher said that the earth _____ around the sun yesterday.

    A. moved   B. was moving

    C. moves   D. is moving

(   ) 2. Charlie _____ here next month.

    A. isn't working   B. doesn't working

    C. isn't going to working   D. won't work

(   ) 3. Will you please say it again? I _____ quite _____ you.

    A. didn't, hear   B. don't, heard

    C. didn't, heard   D. don't, hear

( ) 4. How _____ Mr. Brown _____ to America?

    A. do, go   B. is, go

    C. does, go   D. does, goes

( ) 5. By the time tomorrow, you _____ your homework.

    A. would finish   B. finish

    C. will have finished   D. will finish

( ) 6. There _____ a meeting tomorrow afternoon.

    A. will be going to   B. will going to be

    C. is going to be   D. will go to be

( ) 7. ——Dad, may I go out and play basketball?

    ——_____ you _____ your homework yet?

    A. Have; finished   B. Are; finishing

    C. Did; finish   D. Do; finish

( ) 8. He _____ TV from seven to nine last night.

    A. is watching   B. has watching

    C. has watched   D. was watching

( ) 9. She _____ to bed until she _____ the work.

    A. didn't go; had finished   B. didn't go; have finished

    C. doesn't go; had finished   D. didn't go; finished

( ) 10. ——Mary, could you help me?

    ——Wait a moment. I _____ .

    A. read a book   B. did my homework

    C. was watching TV   D. am cooking dinner.

Supplementary Reading

Everything You Need to Know about Over-The-Counter Drug Abuse

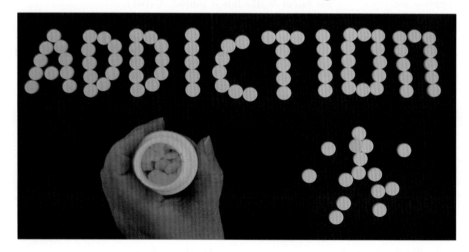

When we think of drug abuse and addiction, we often think of illicit or illegal drugs. But in a May, 2018 article in the FDA Voice blog, Food and Drug Administration Commissioner Scott Gottlieb, M. D. warned of a new pattern of abuse and misuse of over-the-counter (OTC) drugs. Over-the-counter drugs are medications that are available without a prescription and are sold at both at drugstores and supermarkets.

These drugs are safe if used at recommended doses and for recommended time periods. But, just as with illegal drugs and prescription drugs, OTC drugs can be abused. Most common forms of OTC drug abuse include taking the medications in higher doses than recommended, taking them for longer than recommended, and mixing them with other medications to create new products. Even though they are less potent (when taken as recommended) than illicit substances, OTC drugs still pose a risk for addiction.

What Are Some of the Most Commonly Misused OTC Drugs?

· Cough and cold medicines (dextromethorphan or DXM)

· Pain relievers (acetaminophen and ibuprofen)

· Nasal decongestants (pseudoephedrine)

· Motion sickness pills (dimenhydrinate)

· Anti-diarrheal medication (loperamide)

· Diet pills (ephedrine)

· OTC sleep aids/sleeping pills (diphenhydramine)

How Dangerous is the Abuse of OTC Medication?

According to the National Institute on Drug Abuse/ National Institutes of Health, many commonly abused OTC drugs, including cough medicine, anti-diarrhea drugs, motion sickness pills and diet pills, can cause potentially severe and even life-threatening symptoms.

Unfortunately, because these drugs are available over-the-counter, there is often a false sense of safety assumed about them.

People abuse OTC drugs both for recreational use and also inadvertently, by not carefully following dosage recommendations. But they do so at greater risk than they often imagine.

Cough Medicine Abuse

Abuse of cough medicines can cause dizziness, nausea/vomiting, breathing and vision problems, seizures, and anxiety/panic symptoms. When cough medicine products made with DXM are also used with the OTC pain medicine acetaminophen, liver damage can occur.

OTC Pain Medication Abuse

OTC pain medications, like acetaminophen, are generally used for their pain-relieving and fever-reducing properties. Acetaminophen abuse often results from an attempt to treat chronic pain without the use of opioid medication.

Dangers of OTC pain medication medicine abuse: When taken excessively, acetaminophen can severely damage the liver.

Nasal Decongestants (Pseudoephedrine) Abuse

When taken in excessive amounts, nasal decongestant medications can raise blood pressure, increase heart rate to a dangerous level, and cause irregular heartbeat, seizures or hallucinations.

Over-the-Counter Sleeping Pill Abuse

Diphenhydramine can cause constipation, confusion, dizziness and next-day drowsiness, according to the drug's FDA labeling. Another concern, according to a Consumer Reports review is the drug's "hangover effect" —impaired balance, coordination, and driving performance the day after taking the drug, which can increase the risk for falls and accidents.

Abusing OTC Drugs is Risky Business

While the use of over-the-counter drugs may seem, at first glance, to be safe and worry-free, users should beware. The warning of the ancient Greeks, to "do nothing in excess" is certainly appropriate here. Over-the-counter medications are still drugs with powerful and potent active ingredients. Abuse or misuse of these products, such as taking them in excess amounts, can be just as harmful and risky as using illicit drugs.

(535 words)

After-reading Exercises

Task   Decide whether the following statements are true (T) or false (F) according to the text.

(   ) 1. OTC drugs are safe if used at recommended doses and for recommended time periods.

(   ) 2. Because OTC drugs are less potent (when taken as recommended) than illicit substances, they will not pose a risk for addiction.

(   ) 3. When cough medicine products made with DXM are also used with the OTC pain medicine acetaminophen, kidney damage can occur.

(   ) 4. The drug's "hangover effect" is impaired balance, coordination, and driving performance the day after taking the drug, which can increase the risk for falls and accidents.

(   ) 5. The warning of the ancient Greeks, to "do nothing in excess" means you can do anything as much as you wish.

Vocabulary Tips

Prefix "com-, con-"：共同，一起，加强意义。con－用于 c，d，f，g，j，n，q，s，t，v 前，com－的变体。

Example：compassion 同情；compatriot 同胞；commemorate 纪念；comfort 安慰；compress 压缩；contemporary 同时代的；conjoin 联合，结合；conclude 结束，终结；confirm 使坚定；consolidate 巩固，加强；confront 使面对；contribute 贡献，捐献；contaminate 污染，弄脏。

Suffix " –itis"：炎症。

Example：arthritis 关节炎；adenitis 腺炎，淋巴腺炎；adrenalitis 肾上腺炎；allergic rhinitis 过敏性鼻炎；appendicitis 阑尾炎，盲肠炎。

Task　Complete the sentences with the given words.

contaminate	compatriot	consolidate	appendicitis	allergic rhinitis

1. Released wastes heavily _____ the environment and damage crops and human beings.

2. _____ is a diagnosis associated with a group of symptoms affecting the nose.

3. The authorities are trying to _____ security with legality and infrastructure.

4. _____ treatment usually involves surgery to remove the inflamed appendix. Other treatments may be necessary depending on your situation.

5. My dear _____, it is time that we did something for our country.

Proverbs and Sayings

◇It is easy to get a thousand prescriptions, but hard to get one single remedy.

千方易得，一效难求。

◇He who takes medicine and neglects diet wastes the skill of his doctors.

吃药不忌口，枉费大夫手。

◇Nature, time, and patience are the three great physicians.

自然，时间和耐心是三大良医。

题库

Unit **8**

Pharmaceutical Sales and Marketing

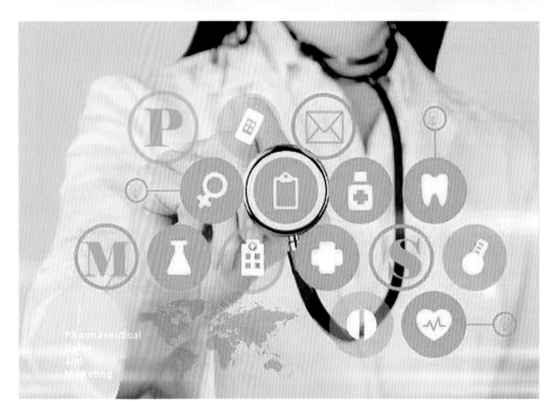

Unit Objectives

After studying this unit, you are expected to:

· master the vocabulary and technical terms related to pharmaceutical sales and marketing;

· understand the development of online pharmaceutical market and major marketing strategies;

· know subjunctive mood correctly.

And you should learn how to:

· communicate with others about introducing people and the agenda of a business conference;

· write a report.

Introduction

Introduction

Sales of pharmaceutical products, which may include medicines, or surgical devices, consumables of any form, machines, and equipment used in surgeries is called pharmaceutical sales. The target audience is doctors of any kind, chemists, and/or purchasing executives in hospitals or pharmacies.

Pharmaceutical marketing, sometimes called medico-marketing or pharma marketing in some countries, is the business of advertising or otherwise promoting the sales of pharmaceuticals or drugs. There is some evidence that marketing practice can affect both patients and the health care profession.

Warming-up

Task   Work in groups. Match the pictures to the proper statements. Then check your answers with your partner.

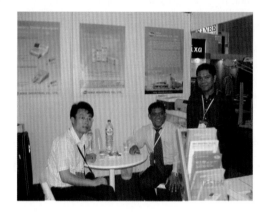

A

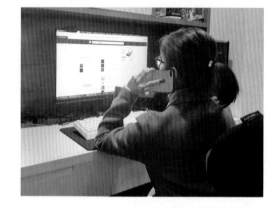

B

C

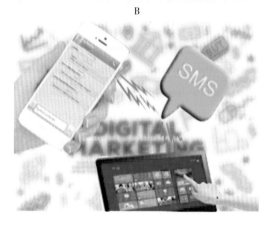

D

(   ) 1. Making business phone calls is considered one of the most effective ways to communicate with one's clients.

(   ) 2. SMS messaging, which stands for short message service marketing, is a strategy that allows businesses to send messages to customers via text.

(   ) 3. An exhibition or a trade fair is held for different companies to exhibit their products and have discussions with potential clients.

(   ) 4. Online marketing tools can be mainly divided into four categories, known as social media tools, SEO (search engine optimization) and ranking tools, content marketing tools and email marketing tools.

Reading A

Chinese Online Pharmacy,
a Bright Way to Sell Drugs

The pharmaceutical industry is one of the major industries in China. The online pharmacy was implemented in China in 2005. In 2008, only 10 online pharmacy shops were permitted to sell drugs at that time. According to China Food and Drug Administration (CFDA), in 2017, 659 online pharmacies obtained the permission. Not only the numbers but also the sales are booming. Figures in Sinohealth's study indicate that the B2C e-pharmacy sales in 2016 increased by 93% year by year and reached almost CNY 28 billion. In 2016, China became the world's second largest pharmaceutical market.

The Chinese Pharmaceutical Market

As the average revenue and the middle class in China are growing, the demand for health care goods and services is getting huge. The older generation wants to save money for their children, so they only spend a little bit of money on themselves. New generations look after themselves much more and they also care more for their family. Spending money on the body or health care is a necessity and normality to them.

The pharmaceutical market was covered by nationwide pharmacy chains. Hospitals were the main place to get drugs and they counted on drug sales for revenue. New rules from the government allow China's e-commerce giants to get a hand in pharmaceuticals by directing prescription drug sales away from hospitals into retail. It aims to enable patients to choose between hospitals and retail pharmacies for prescription drug purchases.

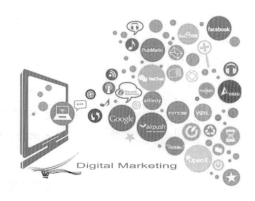

Be Sure to Catch E-pharmacy's Evolution

The fast-growing e-commerce market of China is linked with many new regulations in this area and different new competitors entering the space. The competition in this market is growing, allowing an important place for discount online pharmacy. As this market is on a fast evolution stage, prospects are very rosy. The increase is averaging roughly 30% every year.

E-commerce is also creating opportunity and way for new pharmaceutical brands to sell their products in China. The online pharmacy can promote new brands and new products to customers, creating their needs. With so many discounts online, users will be more attracted and able to spend the time to discover them. Tmall and Jingdong are the most reliable platforms for a major part of Chinese consumers.

The Future of the Pharmaceutical Industry Is Online

The fact to be present on a trusted e-commerce platform reassures consumers to purchase their drugs. With the e-commerce development, Chinese people change their drug purchasing habits. There are different reasons why e-commerce is getting important:

· Because of the very complex distribution chain in China, drug prices used to be very high. Selling on online platforms allows customers to get fairer prices. Information is also more transparent through that way.

· 80% of young Chinese have already done research on the web for their health care. They participate in a discussion on the network and are asking for advice or recommendation of drugs online. They can have access to different propositions and compare them.

· Owing to the high intensity and under pressure work environment in China, Chinese people seek for how to save time and to be more productive. Nowadays, the delivery service in China is very developed. Therefore, to purchase online is as convenient (even more) as going to a drugstore. Customers have no restriction with the time constraint.

(567 words)

Reading A
Words and
Expressions

Words and Expressions			
implement	/ˈimpliment/	vt.	使生效；贯彻；执行；实施
boom	/buːm/	v.	迅速发展；激增；轰鸣
		n.	激增；繁荣
generation	/ˌdʒenəˈreiʃn/	n.	一代；同辈；一代人
necessity	/nəˈsesəti/	n.	必然；必要；必需品
normality	/nɔːˈmæləti/	n.	常态；正常的形势
nationwide	/ˌneiʃnˈwaid/	adj.	全国范围的；全国性的
		adv.	在全国范围内
chain	/tʃein/	n.	链条；连锁商店；一系列
giant	/ˈdʒaiənt/	n.	巨人；巨兽；大公司
		adj.	巨大的；伟大的
retail	/ˈriːteil/	n.	零售
		vt.	零售；零卖；转述
e-commerce	/iːˈkɒmɜːs/	n.	电子商务（同 e-business）
regulation	/ˌregjuˈleiʃn/	n.	章程；规则；规章制度
competitor	/kəmˈpetitə(r)/	n.	竞争者，对手；参赛者
evolution	/ˌiːvəˈluːʃn/	n.	进化；演变；发展
prospect	/ˈprɒspekt/	n.	可能性；希望；前景
roughly	/ˈrʌfli/	adv.	大致；大约；粗糙地
platform	/ˈplætfɔːm/	n.	平台；讲台；站台
reassure	/ˌriːəˈʃʊə(r)/	vt.	使…安心；打消…的疑虑
distribution	/ˌdistriˈbjuːʃn/	n.	经销，分销；分发，分配
transparent	/trænsˈpærənt/	adj.	透明的；清澈的
recommendation	/ˌrekəmenˈdeiʃn/	n.	推荐；介绍；正式建议
proposition	/ˌprɒpəˈziʃn/	n.	提议；建议；任务
restriction	/riˈstrikʃn/	n.	制约因素；限制规定
constraint	/kənˈstreint/	n.	限制；约束
intensity	/inˈtensəti/	n.	强烈；剧烈；强度
count on			预计；指望；依靠
get a hand in			涉足；进军…行业

医药大学堂
WWW.YIYADDXT.COM

续表

participate in	分担；参加
owing to	因为；由于
seek for	寻求；探求；企求
Proper Names	
CNY	人民币（Chinese Yuan）
CFDA	原国家食品药品监督管理总局（China Food and Drug Administration），现国家药品监督管理局（National Medical Products Administration，NMPA）
Sinohealth	中康咨询，医药行业综合数据平台
B2C	商对客电子商务模式（Business-to-Consumer）
Tmall	天猫，综合性购物网站
Jingdong	京东，综合网上购物商城

📖 Notes

1. In 2016, China became the world's second largest pharmaceutical market.

2016 年，中国成为世界第二大医药市场。

"the world's second largest"，序数词加形容词最高级，意为"第几大"。

e. g. The US has the third largest population in the world.

美国是世界第三大人口大国。

2. New rules from the government allow China's e-commerce giants to get a hand in pharmaceuticals by directing prescription drug sales away from hospitals into retail.

政府的新规定允许中国电商巨头涉足医药领域，将处方药销售从医院转向零售。

"by directing prescription drug sales …"为介词加现在分词短语，用作方式状语。

e. g. He finished the project ahead of schedule by working day and night.

他日夜工作，使项目得以提前完成。

3. The fast-growing e-commerce market of China is linked with many new regulations in this area and different new competitors entering the space.

中国电子商务市场的快速增长与该领域的许多新规定以及不同的新竞争者进入该领域有关。

"be linked with"意为"与……相关联"。

e. g. While the disease can be linked with lifestyle, it has genetic causes too.

虽然这种疾病可能与生活方式有关，但它也有遗传原因。

"entering the space"为现在分词短语作后置定语，相当于定语从句"who/which enter the space"。

e. g. They built a highway leading into the mountains.

他们修建了一条通往山区的高速公路。

4. As this market is on a fast evolution stage, prospects are very rosy.

由于市场正处于快速发展阶段，前景非常乐观。

"be on…stage"意为"处于……阶段"。

e. g. At present, China is still on the initial stage of socialism.

目前，中国仍处于社会主义初级阶段。

5. Therefore, to purchase online is as convenient（even more）as going to a drugstore.

因此，网上购物和去药店一样方便（甚至更方便）。

"as…as…" 意为 "和……一样……"。

e. g. This film is not as interesting as that one.

这部电影不如那部有趣。

After-reading Exercises

Task 1   Answer the following questions according to the text.

1. When did China become the world's second largest pharmaceutical market and what was the total sales then?

_____

2. Why is the demand for health care goods and services getting huge?

_____

3. What is the purpose of the government's new rules allowing China's e-commerce giants to get a hand in the pharmaceuticals?

_____

4. How does the fast-growing e-commerce market benefit manufacturers in China?

_____

5. What kind of influence does e-commerce have on drug prices?

_____

Task 2   Match the words（1-10）to the Chinese meanings（a-j）.

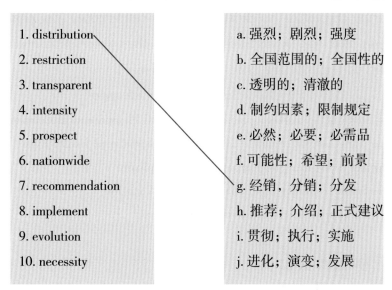

1. distribution	a. 强烈；剧烈；强度
2. restriction	b. 全国范围的；全国性的
3. transparent	c. 透明的；清澈的
4. intensity	d. 制约因素；限制规定
5. prospect	e. 必然；必要；必需品
6. nationwide	f. 可能性；希望；前景
7. recommendation	g. 经销，分销；分发
8. implement	h. 推荐；介绍；正式建议
9. evolution	i. 贯彻；执行；实施
10. necessity	j. 进化；演变；发展

Task 3   Fill in each blank with the proper form of the word or phrase given in brackets.

1. Health care service must _____ with China's economic development.（evolution）

2. The conference focused on the _____ and importance of the modernization of Chinese

medicine. （necessary）

3. _____ of food and medical supplies is going ahead using a network of local volunteers. （distribute）

4. With the fast development of e-business, the pharmaceutical _____ have all entered this new industry. （giant）

5. They signed a secret deal with their major _____ . （compete）

Task 4   Translate the following sentences into English using the words or phrases you have learned in this unit.

1. 根据原国家食品药品监督管理总局的数据，2017 年有 659 家网上药店获得许可。（online）

_____

2. 医院是获取药品的主要场所，他们依靠药品销售获得收入。（count on）

_____

3. 其目的是使患者在购买处方药时可在医院和零售药店之间选择。（retail）

_____

4. 电子商务也为新的医药品牌在中国销售产品创造了机会和途径。（opportunity）

_____

5. 对于大多数中国消费者来说，天猫和京东是最为可靠的平台。（reliable）

_____

Listening & Speaking

Listening &
Speaking
Task 1

Task 1   During the coffee break at a business conference, Ms. Zhang Yang and Mr. Wang Jun meet Mr. David Smith. Listen to the conversation and decide whether the following statements are true （T） or false （F） .

I'd Like to Introduce My Colleague.

（   ） 1. David Smith is the marketing manager from ABC Pharmaceutical Company.

（   ） 2. Zhang Yang met Mr. Smith at 2019 Beijing International Health Expo.

（   ） 3. Wang Jun is the marketing manager from Sinopharm.

（   ） 4. David Smith is introduced to Zhang Yang by Wang Jun.

（   ） 5. The three people meet at a business conference.

📖 **Notes**

1. Sinopharm   中国医药集团。

2. London International Health Expo.   伦敦国际医疗展。

Listening &
Speaking
Task 2

Task 2   Robert and Mike are talking about tomorrow's general meeting. Listen to the conversation and choose the best answer to each question you hear.

What's on the Cards for Tomorrow's General Meeting?

（   ） 1. Who is going to give a rundown on the company's most recent sales figures?

A. Sales director   B. A sales representative

C. Sales manager   D. Marketing manager

(   ) 2. Why is everyone requested to attend the meeting?

A. Because new tasks are going to be assigned

B. Because the recent sales is not as good as last year's

C. Because it will be important for company's near-term future

D. Because it is the company's rule

(   ) 3. Who will be responsible for reminding everyone of the conference?

A. Robert

B. Robert's secretary

C. Mike

D. Someone from the marketing department

(   ) 4. Which department will send someone to give their viewpoint on the sales results?

A. The marketing department   B. The logistics department C

C. The financial department   D. The HR department

(   ) 5. Which of the following statements is correct?

A. The general meeting will be held next week.

B. Not everyone is required to attend the meeting.

C. The marketing department is in charge of the meeting.

D. Someone from the marketing department needs to hurry since time is limited.

📖 Notes

1. What's on the cards for tomorrow's general meeting?

明天的大会有什么安排?

"on the cards": 在安排表上。

2. rundown   简要介绍，简单叙述。

3. I hope they will be able to prepare something on such a short notice.

我希望他们能在这么短时间内准备好一些必要的资料。

"on such a short notice": 在这么短时间内。

Task 3   Pharmacoeconomics is new in the field of economics. Listen to the following passage and fill in the blanks with what you hear.

"Pharmacoeconomics" is a new word; but economic interest in drug and other treatments of _____ 1 _____ problems is much older. _____ 2 _____ about what treatments should be appropriate within a health care system have always been influenced by the resources _____ 3 _____ to pay for them. Pharmacoeconomics can be _____ 4 _____ as the branch of economics that uses cost-benefit, cost-effectiveness, cost-minimization, cost-of-illness and cost-utility analyses to compare pharmaceutical _____ 5 _____ and treatment strategies.

Listening &

Speaking

Task 3

Task 4   The marketing manager, A, and his/her secretary, B, are at the airport to welcome their client, C. Work in groups and practice making the conversations with your partners according to what you hear in the Listening part.

Partner A	Partner B	Partner C
Greet C.		Greet A and thank for the invitation.
Introduce B.	Greet C.	Greet B.
	Ask about the trip.	Talk about the trip.
Inform C of the business conference.	Give a detailed introduction of the agenda.	Ask about the agenda of the conference.
Send C to the hotel.	Say goodbye.	Express thanks and say goodbye.

Reading B

Bayer Marketing Mix（4Ps）Strategy

Marketing Mix of Bayer analyzes the brand/company which covers 4Ps（Product, Price, Place, Promotion）and explains the Bayer marketing strategy. As of 2020, there are several marketing strategies like product/service innovation, marketing investment, customer experience etc., which have helped the brand grow.

Marketing strategy helps companies achieve business goals and objectives, and marketing mix（4Ps）is the widely used framework to define the strategies. Following is the 4Ps strategy elaborating the product, pricing, distribution and advertising strategies used by Bayer.

Bayer Product Strategy

Bayer offers a wide range of products to its customers. There are major brands which form the part of Bayer's marketing mix product portfolio strategy. These products help us to find the solutions that pose a great challenge to us. They are mainly divided into four categories. Pharmaceutical category includes products that are prescribed for women health care, cardiology, oncology and haematology. Bayer's top selling products include Kogenate, Betaseron, Trasylol and Cipro. Another category for Bayer products is consumer health products. These consist of main products that are non-prescribed under the category dermatology, allergy, cough and cold, foot care and sun care. Apart from these two, third category

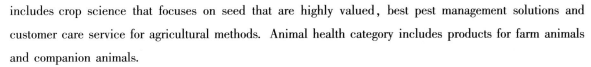

includes crop science that focuses on seed that are highly valued, best pest management solutions and customer care service for agricultural methods. Animal health category includes products for farm animals and companion animals.

Bayer Price / Pricing Strategy

Pricing plays an important role in pharmaceutical industry. Bayer has always focused on quality products. To maintain that quality, price becomes an important factor. It has always followed a competition-based marketing mix pricing strategy. For most of its products, the prices are similar to the prices of its competitors' products. But, the differentiating factor is the quality that they never compromised. They have their own sites for procurement. Thus, it reduces costs, smoothens delivery system as well as they can follow security and environmental securities as per the set global standards.

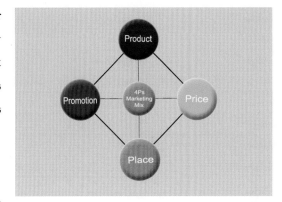

Bayer Place & Distribution Strategy

Place management is very important for Bayer. This ensures that goods and services are available in right time at right place. This helps the smooth flow of materials in the distribution channels. They are very peculiar when it comes to choose suppliers for their products. They have defined their own code of conduct named Bayer's supply code of conduct for suppliers. Environmental, social and governance standards decide whether to continue with existing suppliers or not. Now, these suppliers transfer the products to various certified retailers and finally through retailers, these products reach to customers.

Bayer Promotion & Advertising Strategy

Bayer founded its own sporting club named Bayer 04 Leverkusen. It is pretty famous for being a football club, but it has also participated in various other sports such as volleyball, boxing, basketball and athletics. In Germany, it is one of the largest sports club. The company also sponsors other clubs such as Dormagen, Wuppertal and many others. The company has presence in various social media platforms such as Facebook, Twitter, YouTube, LinkedIn, Instagram, etc. They have also introduced E-cards that can be sent to your dear ones free of cost through Bayer's world. This covers the marketing mix of Bayer.

(543 words)

Words and Expressions			
framework	/ˈfreimwɜːk/	n.	构架，框架；机制
elaborate	/iˈlæbəreit/	vt.	详细阐述；精心制作
objective	/əbˈdʒektiv/	n.	目标；目的
pricing	/ˈpraisiŋ/	n.	定价；计价
		vt.	给…定价；标价
portfolio	/pɔːtˈfəuliəu/	n.	组合；投资组合
cardiology	/ˌkɑːdiˈɒlədʒi/	n.	心脏病学
oncology	/ɒŋˈkɒlədʒi/	n.	肿瘤学
haematology	/ˌhiːməˈtɒlədʒi/	n.	血液学

续表

dermatology	/ˌdɜːməˈtɒlədʒi/	n.	皮肤病学
pest	/pest/	n.	害虫；讨厌的人
companion	/kəmˈpæniən/	n.	伴侣；同伴；陪伴
factor	/ˈfæktə(r)] /	n.	因素；要素；因子
differentiate	/ˌdifəˈrenʃieit/	vt.	区分；区别；区别对待
compromise	/ˈkɒmprəmaiz/	vt.	妥协，让步；违背
procurement	/prəˈkjuəmənt/	n.	采购，购买
smoothen	/ˈsmuːðən/	vt.	使平滑；使平和
available	/əˈveiləbl/	adj.	可获得的；有空的
peculiar	/piˈkjuːliə(r)] /	adj.	奇怪的；不寻常的
code	/kəʊd/	n.	密码；代码；行为准则
governance	/ˈgʌvənəns/	n.	统治；管理；治理
certified	/ˈsɜːtifaid/	adj.	被证实的；有保证的
channel	/ˈtʃænl/	n.	频道；途径；渠道
presence	/ˈprezns/	n.	出席；在场；存在

Proper Names

Bayer	拜耳，德国著名医药产业集团
Kogenate	拜科奇，重组抗血友病因子
Betaseron	倍泰龙，治疗多发性硬化症药物
Trasylol	抑肽酶
Cipro	齐普罗，盐酸环丙沙星制剂
Bayer 04 Leverkusen	勒沃库森足球俱乐部
Dormagen	多尔马根手球俱乐部
Wuppertal	伍珀塔尔足球俱乐部
Facebook	脸书，社交网络服务网站
Twitter	推特，社交及微博客服务网站
YouTube	油管，视频网站
LinkedIn	领英，职场社交招聘平台
Instagram	照片墙，图片分享社交应用

After-reading Exercises

Task 1   Read the passage and choose the correct answer to each question.

(   ) 1. Which of the following is not Bayer Marketing Mix (4Ps)？

A. Product strategy   B. Price strategy

C. Promotion strategy   D. Public relations strategy

(   ) 2. Bayer's main products can be divided into the following four categories except _____ .

A. pharmaceutical category   B. consumer health products

C. beauty products   D. animal health category

(   ) 3. Which of the following does not belong to the benefits of having their own sites for procurement?

  A. Reduce costs

  B. Reduce work hours

  C. Smoothen delivery system

  D. Follow security and environmental securities

( ) 4. Which factor may decide whether to continue with existing suppliers or not?

  A. Low cost

  B. Diverse products

  C. Delivery on time

  D. Environmental, social and governance standards

( ) 5. Which of the following sporting clubs is not sponsored by Bayer?

  A. FC Bayern München   B. Bayer 04 Leverkusen

  C. Dormagen   D. Wuppertal

Task 2　Translate the following sentences into Chinese.

1. Marketing strategy helps companies achieve business goalsand objectives, and marketing mix (4Ps) is the widely used framework to define the strategies.

  _____

2. Apart from these two, third category includes crop science that focuses on seed that are highly valued, best pest management solutions and customer care service for agricultural methods.

  _____

3. Thus, it reduces costs, smoothens delivery system as well as they can follow security and environmental securities as per the set global standards.

  _____

4. Environmental, social and governance standards decide whether to continue with existing suppliers or not.

  _____

5. It is pretty famous for being a football club, but it has also participated in various other sports such as volleyball, boxing, basketball and athletics.

  _____

Practical Writing

Report

  报告是下级向上级汇报工作、反应情况、提出意见或建议的一种应用文。无论是哪一种报告，在写作上都要遵循以下几点：

  1. 明确报告的读者，分析其需要。

  2. 语气要客观、真实。

  3. 运用叙述、说明等正式表达方式，不使用乞使、请求等表达方式。

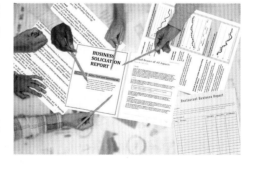

Sample

Report on College Students' Reading Habits

This report aims to discover college students' reading habits.

The survey was conducted among 16 college students at Peking University by means of questionnaire on February 16th. The questionnaire dealt with students' reading habits and reading frequency.

As can be seen, 81% of the students regularly read academic books, while 44% regularly read academic journals. Nothing else is read often by 10% of the students. In regard to students' extracurricular reading, 55% regularly read newspaper or magazines, while 34% sometimes read fiction and 12% never read.

We may draw a conclusion from the data that college students presumably allocate little time for general reading, and most of their reading time is spent on books and journals on their own subject.

Li Ming

报告通常包含以下项目：

1. 标题（Title）：标题要准确、客观概括报告的内容，一般使用"Report on …"，如：

Report on Improving Training Methods.

Report on the Proposed Incentive Scheme.

2. 导言（Introduction）：导言部分应扼要说明一下报告的写作背景和主旨。以下是导言部分的常见句型：

The report examines/ explains…

The purpose of this report is to…investigate / evaluate / study…

The aim of this report is to…analyze / summarize / assess…

3. 调查结果（Findings）：报告的调查结果是结论和建议的依据。以下是这部分的常见句型：

The findings of the… indicate / show that…

It was proposed / found / felt / discovered that…

4. 结论（Conclusions）：报告的结论部分是对调查结果进行总结和解释，必要时可提出建议。以下是这部分的常见句型：

We may draw a conclusion that…

To conclude, we can see that (the best way/solution is) …

We strongly recommend that…

Task   Barrie Watson is going to write a workshop report on Effective Team Leadership. Complete the following report with key sentence patterns and the information given below in Chinese.

研讨会主要内容：

1. 总结最近的团队领导力研讨会，并提出适当的行动建议。

2. 建议公司确保团队领导能胜任符合公司期望的关键性任务。

3. 建议公司设立一个评估中心（assessment center），对团队领导进行评估，以确保他们具备有效团队领导的特征。

Report on Effective Team Leadership

_____

_____

_____ the team leaders had different understandings of their roles based on the assessment during the workshop. Having identified the different possible approaches to each key task, the company was able to select which was most appropriate in terms of skills and behavior required.

_____. Therefore, we strongly recommend the company should immediately set up _____ .

Barrie Watson

Grammar Tips

英语中共有三种语气：

1. 陈述语气：用来陈述事实、提出想法。

2. 祈使语气：用来提出请求、命令等。

3. 虚拟语气：用来表示说话人的主观愿望、建议、命令等，有时是非真实的假设，或是不可能实现的与事实相反的愿望。

Subjunctive Mood

类别	用法	
if 引导的条件状语从句	与现在事实相反	从句：一般过去时（be 用 were） 主句：should / would / could / might + 动词原形
	e. g. If he were here, he would help us.	
	与过去事实相反	从句：过去完成时 主句：should / would / could / might + have + 过去分词
	e. g. If I had been free, I would have given you a call.	
	与将来事实相反	从句：一般过去时 / should + 动词原形 / were + 不定式 主句：should / would / could / might + 动词原形
	e. g. If it should rain tomorrow, we would not visit the factory.	
其他状语从句	as if 引导的状语从句中动词用一般过去时或过去完成时	
	e. g. They are talking as if they had been friends for years.	
	for fear that（唯恐），in case（以防），lest（以防）引导的目的状语从句中，谓语动词用 should + 动词原形	
	e. g. He started earlier lest he should be late.	

续表

类别	用法
宾语从句	wish 后的从句中分别用一般过去时、过去完成时或 should / would + 动词原形
	e. g. I wish I could be a pop singer.
	demand / suggest / order / insist 等表示命令、建议、愿望等动词后的从句中用（should）+ 动词原形
	e. g. He suggested that we (should) not change our mind.
主语从句	在 It is necessary / important / that…, It is suggested / requested / demanded that…等主语从句中，谓语动词用（should）+ 动词原形
	e. g. It is necessary that we (should) take exercises to keep us healthy.
表语从句	The + suggestion / recommendation / request is that…等表语从句中，谓语动词用（should）+ 动词原形
	e. g. The order is that each doctor (should) return to the hospital right away.
其他句型	It is (high) time that…后的主语从句中动词用一般过去时或 should + 动词原形
	e. g. It's high time that we finished the sales meeting.
	would rather 后的从句中动词用一般过去时或过去完成时
	e. g. I would rather you hadn't been ill.
	If only 句型中动词常用一般过去时或过去完成时，表示强烈愿望
	e. g. If only he had come five minutes earlier.

Task 1 Fill in each of the following blanks with the proper form of the given words.

1. The manager recommended that all sales people _____ on-site training. (take)

2. It was proposed by all attendants that John _____ as chairman of the pharmaceutical company. (appoint)

3. It is generally thought important to a man that he _____ himself. (know)

4. If you had been with us, our excitement _____. (understand)

5. He talks about Rome as if he _____ there before. (be)

6. You stayed up the whole night for the new product launch. It is high time you _____ to bed. (go)

7. If this _____ again, they would have to bear the consequences. (happen)

8. Had it not been for our manager standing up for him, he _____. (have to leave)

9. She wasn't in good health, otherwise she _____ harder. (work)

10. The general manager has rejected all the workers' demand that their monthly salaries _____ by 10 percent. (raise)

Task 2 Choose the best answer to complete each sentence according to the Sentence Component.

(   ) 1. The guard at the gate insisted that everybody _____ the rules.

    A. obeys   B. obey

    C. would obey   D. to obey

(   ) 2. If all the team members had tried their best, they _____ the bid.

    A. will win   B. had won

  C. should win   D. would have won

( ) 3. How I wish I _____ you yesterday!

  A. saw   B. see

  C. had seen   D. were to see

( ) 4. Without electricity human life _____ quite different today.

  A. will be   B. is

  C. would be   D. would have been

( ) 5. The teacher demanded that the exam _____ before eleven.

  A. must finish   B. would be finished

  C. be finished   D. must be finished

( ) 6. My suggestion was that the meeting _____ off till next week.

  A. to put   B. be put

  C. should put   D. be putting

( ) 7. Had you listened to the doctor, you _____ all right now.

  A. are   B. were

  C. would be   D. would have been

( ) 8. He treated me as if I _____ his own son.

  A. were   B. am

  C. was   D. would be

( ) 9. If it hadn't been for the storm, the delivery _____ delayed.

  A. wouldn't be   B. won't be

  C. wouldn't have been   D. shouldn't be

( ) 10. If only he had told us the truth in the first place, things _____ so wrong.

  A. should go   B. would have gone

  C. would go   D. wouldn't have gone

Supplementary Reading

Pharmaceutical Industry

Sales and Marketing

Background

  Pharmaceutical industry sales and marketing indicates the business of promoting pharmaceuticals both for the clinical aspects of the product and gaining market share. Some aspects focus on the capability to analyze the needs of a given market and others on developing communications about specific therapies and products.

  Pharmacists in this field follow guidelines and rules supported throughout the industry. PhRMA——the Pharmaceutical Research and Manufacturers of America——created a code several years ago for sales and marketing personnel to follow. The information below gives a glimpse of the depth of the PhRMA Code:

1. Prohibits company sales representatives from providing restaurant meals to health care professionals, but allows them to provide occasional meals in health care professionals' offices in conjunction with informational presentations.

2. Includes new provisions requiring companies to ensure their representatives are sufficiently trained about applicable laws, regulations, and industry codes of practice and ethics.

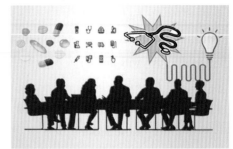

3. Provides that each company will state its intentions to abide by the Code and that company CEOs and compliance officers will certify each year that they have processes in place to comply.

4. Includes more detailed standards regarding the independence of continuing medical education.

5. Provides additional guidance and restrictions for speaking and consulting arrangements with health care professionals.

PhRMA Code——revised guidelines 2009

In addition to the traditional sales calls, there has been an emergence of new communication vehicles used. Social media technologies are changing the pharmaceutical marketing process. The opportunities to work with multiple media vehicles have opened new marketing strategies and sales initiatives.

What aspects of the job are most appealing?

One of the most appealing aspects of these roles, cited by 27% of pharmacist respondents, was related to the impact they can have on patients. For many, this is an indirect benefit of the role. The same percentage also indicated that an appealing aspect was working and collaborating with other health care professionals (i. e., pharmacists, physicians, nurses, or others).

One respondent stated, "Love interaction with clinicians throughout the health care market." Another added enjoyment in "working with pharmacists and nurses to improve patient safety and save costs."

Thirteen percent cited the work environment as one of the most appealing aspects of their role. Many corporate offices are modern and have amenities that can be used by employees. One commented on working in a "very nice work environment."

What aspects of the job are least appealing?

Bureaucracy and politics were both cited by 18% of pharmacists as among the least appealing aspects of their role. These pharmacists are very satisfied with the work they perform, but one respondent stated finding the "administrative work and the politics of a large corporation" as a least appealing aspect of the role. Administrative paperwork and travel were cited by 9% of the respondents. One respondent indicated not liking the "travel and being away from clinical practice."

(490 words)

After-reading Exercises

Task Decide whether the following statements are true (T) or false (F) according to the text.

( ) 1. The PhRMA Code allows company sales representatives to provide restaurant meals to health care professionals.

( ) 2. Companies are required to ensure their representatives are sufficiently trained about applicable laws, regulations, and industry codes of practice and ethics.

(　) 3. The opportunities to work with people have opened new marketing strategies and sales initiatives.

(　) 4. One of the most appealing aspects of working in sales and marketing industry is that they can travel a lot.

(　) 5. Some insiders don't like administrative work and the politics of a large corporation.

Vocabulary Tips

Root "onco-, oncus-, oncho-": 肿瘤，块。来自希腊语 onkos，大块，肿块，引申词义肿瘤。

Example: oncology 肿瘤学；adenoncus 腺肿大；arthroncus 关节肿大；blepharoncus 睑瘤；glossoncus 舌肿；gonyoncus 膝瘤。

Root "h（a）emo-, h（a）emato-": 血，血液。

Example: haematology 血液学血液病学；hemodiagnosis 验血诊断；anhematosis 血液生成不足；hemocircular 血液循环；hemorrhage 出血。

Root "dermat-": 皮肤。源于希腊语或拉丁语 dermat，derma/demat 皮肤。

Example: dermatology 皮肤病学；dermatologist 皮肤病学家；dermatitis 皮炎；hypoderm 皮下组织。

Task　Complete the sentences with the given words.

hypodermic	hemodiagnosis	hemorrhage	dermatitis	arthroncus

1. Not eating enough of vitamins can result in problems such as scurvy（坏血病），_____ or dry, scaly skin（鳞状皮肤）.

2. The _____ in Harry's knee seemed to be the result of an accumulation of fluid under the knee cap.

3. You might run out of platelets（血小板）before you can control the _____ .

4. As he reached over, Mary slid a _____ syringe（注射器）into his left arm.

5. _____ is diagnosis by means of examination of the blood.

Proverbs and Sayings

◇The wise will not rely on medicine for keeping their health.

　智者从不依赖药物来维持健康。

◇The best doctors are Dr. Diet, Dr. Quite and Dr. Merryman.

　最好的医生是饮食、宁静和快乐。

◇Prevention is better than cure.

　预防胜于治疗。

题库

医药大学堂
WWW.YIYAODXT.COM

PPT

Unit **9**

Medicines Regulation

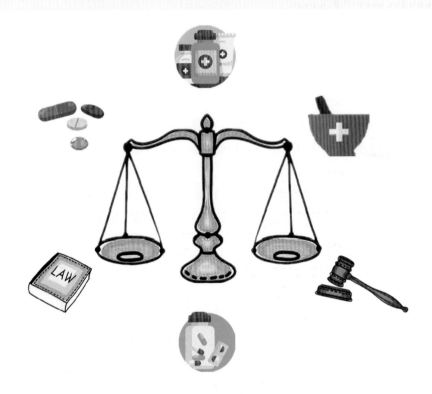

Unit Objectives

After studying this unit, you are expected to:

· master the vocabulary and technical terms related to Medicines Regulation;

· know Medicines Regulation and Health Insurance;

· understand Concord.

And you should learn how to:

· communicate with others about the food contamination and food poisoning;

· write a business letter.

Introduction

Medicines regulation incorporates several mutually reinforcing activities all aimed at promoting and protecting public health. These activities vary from country to country in scope and implementation, but generally include the following functions:

· Licensing of the manufacture, import, export, distribution, promotion and advertising of medicines.

· Assessing the safety, efficacy and quality of medicines, and issuing marketing authorization for individual products.

· Inspecting and surveillance of manufacturers, importers, wholesalers and dispensers of medicines.

· Controlling and monitoring the quality of medicines on the market.

· Controlling promotion and advertising of medicines.

· Monitoring safety of marketed medicines including collecting and analyzing adverse reaction reports.

· Providing independent information on medicines to professionals and the public.

Warming-up

Task **Work in groups. Match the logos to the proper statements. Then check your answers with your partner.**

A

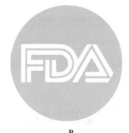

B

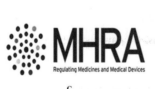

C

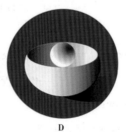

D

(　) 1. The European Medicines Agency (EMA) is responsible for the scientific evaluation, supervision and safety monitoring of medicines developed by pharmaceutical companies for use in the EU.

(　) 2. The UK's regulator of medicines, medical devices and blood components for transfusion, is responsible for ensuring their safety, quality and effectiveness.

( ) 3. The Food and Drug Administration is responsible for protecting the public health in USA by assuring the safety, efficacy, and security of human and veterinary drugs, biological products, medical devices, nation's food supply, cosmetics, and products that emit radiation.

( ) 4. The Ministry of Health, Labour and Welfare in Japan provides regulations on maximum residue limits for agricultural chemicals in foods, basic food and drug regulations, standards for foods, food additives, etc.

Reading A

Reading A

Medicines Regulation

History of Medicines Regulation

Medicines are perhaps as old as mankind and the concepts how their quality has to be ensured has evolved gradually over the time. It took until 1540 when in England the manufacture of medicines was subjected to supervision under the Apothecaries, Wares, Drugs and Stuffs Act. This could be seen as the start of pharmaceutical inspections. History of Pharmacopoeias, the official books of drug quality standards, probably dates back to one of the proclamations of the Salerno Medical Edict issued by Fredrick II of Sicily (1240). The first Pharmacopoeias as we know them today started to appear in Europe from 16th century e. g. the first Spanish Pharmacopoeia was issued in 1581.

The modern medicines regulation started only after breakthrough progress in the 19th century life sciences, especially in chemistry, physiology and pharmacology, which laid a solid foundation for the modern drug research and development and started to flourish after the Second World War.

Drug Registration

Registration of drugs, also known as product licensing or marketing authorization, is an essential element of drug regulation. All drugs that are marketed, distributed and used in the country should be registered by the national competent regulatory authority.

Drug regulation should include the scientific evaluation of products before registration, to ensure that all marketed pharmaceutical products meet the criteria of safety, efficacy and quality. These criteria are applicable to all medicines including biological products (including vaccines, blood products, monoclonal antibodies, cell and tissue therapies) and herbal medicines.

Why Regulating Drugs?

Drugs are not ordinary consumers' products. In most instances, consumers are not in a position to make decisions about when to use drugs, which drugs to use, how to use them and to weigh potential benefits against risks as no medicine is completely safe. Professional advice from either prescribers or dispensers is needed in making these decisions. Thus, Governments need to establish strong national regulatory authorities (NRAs), to ensure that the manufacture, trade and use of medicines are regulated effectively. In broad terms the mission of NRAs is to protect and promote public health.

What Makes Medicines Regulation Effective?

Medicines regulation demands the application of sound medical, scientific and technical knowledge and skills, and operates within a legal framework. Regulatory functions involve interactions with various stakeholders (e.g. manufacturers, traders, consumers, health professionals, researchers and governments) whose economic, social and political motives may differ, making implementation of regulation both politically and technically challenging. All medicines must meet three criteria: be of good quality,

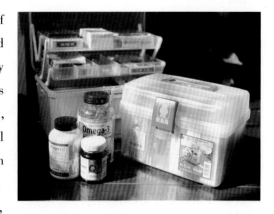

safe and effective. The judgments about medicines quality, safety and efficacy should be based on solid science.

(430 words)

Reading A
Words and
Expressions

Words and Expressions			
drug	/drʌg/	n.	药；毒品
stuff	/stʌf/	n.	东西；材料；填充物
pharmacopoeia	/ˌfɑːməkəˈpiːə/	n.	药典
breakthrough	/ˈbreikθruː/	n.	突破
foundation	/faʊnˈdeiʃn/	n.	基础；地基
flourish	/ˈflʌriʃ/	v.	繁荣，茂盛
element	/ˈelimənt/	n.	元素；要素；原理
market	/ˈmɑːkit/	vt.	在市场上出售
distribute	/diˈstribjuːt/	vt.	分配；把……分类
competent	/ˈkɒmpitənt/	adj.	胜任的；有能力的
professional	/prəˈfeʃənl/	adj.	专业的；职业的
dispenser	/diˈspensə(r)/	n.	药剂师；施与者
broad	/brɔːd/	adj.	宽的，辽阔的
mission	/ˈmiʃn/	n.	使命，任务
interaction	/ˌintərˈækʃn/	n.	相互作用，相互影响
motive	/ˈməʊtiv/	n.	动机，目的
differ	/ˈdifə(r)/	vt.	使……相异；使……不同
implementation	/ˌimplimenˈteiʃn/	n.	实现；履行

Proper Names	
the Apothecaries Wares, Drugs and Stuffs Act	《药剂师货品、药品和物品法》
the proclamations of the Salerno Medical Edict	《萨莱诺医学法令》
Fredrick Ⅱ of Sicily	西西里的弗雷德里克二世
Spanish Pharmacopoeia	《西班牙药典》
national regulatory authorities (NRAs)	国家监管部门

医药大学堂
WWW.YIYAODXT.COM

📖 Notes

1. It took until 1540 when in England the manufacture of medicines was subjected to supervision under the Apothecaries Wares, Drugs and Stuffs Act.

直到 1540 年，英格兰的药品生产才受到《药剂师货品、药品和物品法》的监管。

"until（或 till）" 意为 "直到……时"，表示的是一段时间的终点。

e. g. It was not until 1911 that the first of the vitamins was identified.

直到 1911 年才发现了第一种维生素。

"be subject to" 意为 "受支配，从属于"。

e. g. Prices may be subject to alteration.

价格可能会受变更影响。

2. The modern medicines regulation started only after breakthrough progress in the 19th century life sciences, especially in chemistry, physiology and pharmacology, which laid a solid foundation for the modern drug research and development and started to flourish after the second World War.

现代药物监管是在 19 世纪生命科学特别是化学、生理学和药理学取得突破性进展后开始的，为现代药物研发奠定了坚实的基础，并在第二次世界大战后开始蓬勃发展。

"which" 引导的非限定性定语从句，修饰主语 "the modern medicines regulation"。

e. g. He may have acute appendicitis, which caused his right lower abdominal pain, nausea and vomiting.

他可能得了急性阑尾炎，导致右下腹痛、恶心和呕吐。

3. Drug regulation should include the scientific evaluation of products before registration, to ensure that all marketed pharmaceutical products meet the criteria of safety, efficacy and quality.

药品监管应包括注册前对产品进行科学评估，以确保所有上市的药品都安全、有效并符合质量标准。

"to ensure that…" 不定式在句子中作目的状语，"that…" 引导宾语从句。

e. g. We tried to ensure that everyone got a fair deal.

我们曾尽力保证每个人都受到公平待遇。

4. In most instances, consumers are not in a position to make decisions about when to use drugs, which drugs to use, how to use them and to weigh potential benefits against risks as no medicine is completely safe.

在大多数情况下，由于没有一种药物是绝对安全的，消费者无法决定何时使用药物、使用哪些药物、如何使用药物以及权衡潜在的益处和风险。

"in a position to" 意为 "能够，可以"。

e. g. I am not in a position to comment.

我不便发表评论。

"… when to do…which to do… how to do…"，不定式在句中充当介词 about 的宾语。"介词/动词 + 疑问词 + to do" 是不定式做宾语的常见结构，可以在连接代词（what，who，which）或连接副词（how，when，where）及连词 whether 后面接一个带 to 的不定式，可以将这种结构看成是连接词引导的宾语从句的简略形式。

e. g. I wonder who to invite.（= I wonder who I should invite.）

我想知道该邀请谁。

5. Regulatory functions involve interactions with various stakeholders (e. g. manufacturers, traders,

consumers, health professionals, researchers and governments) whose economic, social and political motives may differ, making implementation of regulation both politically and technically challenging.

监管职能涉及与各种利益攸关方（例如制造商、贸易商、消费者、卫生专业人员、研究人员和政府）的相互作用，这些利益攸关方的经济、社会和政治动机可能不同，这使得监管的实施在政治上和技术上都具有挑战性。

"involve…with"意为"涉及，牵涉"。

e. g. Don't involve you with those people.

别与那些人混在一起。

"whose"引导定语从句，意为"……的……"，它所指代的先行词可以是人或事物，在具体语境中灵活处理。它引导的定语从句修饰它的先行词，同时它本身在从句中做定语。

e. g. He lives in a room whose window faces north.

他住在一个窗户面朝北的房间里。

After-reading Exercises

Task 1   Answer the following questions according to the text.

1. When did the first pharmacopoeia appear in Europe?

_____

2. What has facilitated the development of modern medicines regulation?

_____

3. What is the most important element of medicines regulation?

_____

4. What does the effective drug regulation demand?

_____

5. What criteria must all medicines meet?

_____

Task 2   Match the words（1-10）to the Chinese meanings（a-j）.

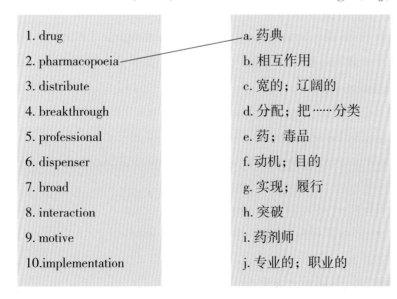

1. drug	a. 药典
2. pharmacopoeia	b. 相互作用
3. distribute	c. 宽的；辽阔的
4. breakthrough	d. 分配；把……分类
5. professional	e. 药；毒品
6. dispenser	f. 动机；目的
7. broad	g. 实现；履行
8. interaction	h. 突破
9. motive	i. 药剂师
10.implementation	j. 专业的；职业的

Task 3　Fill in each blank with the proper form of the word or phrase given in brackets.

1. The new edition of the _____ marks a new stage in China's pharmaceutical standards. (pharmacology)

2. The money will go to the San Francisco AIDS _____ . (foundational)

3. Few businesses are _____ in the present economic climate. (flourish)

4. They studied the geographical _____ of the disease. (distribute)

5. Leadership is about the ability to _____ change. (implementation)

Task 4　Translate the following sentences into English using the words or phrases you have learned in this unit.

1. 凡在国内销售、分销和使用的药品，必须经国家管理机构注册。(distribute; the national regulatory authority)

_____

2. 药品监管应包括注册前对产品进行科学评估，以确保所有上市的药品都安全、有效并符合质量标准。(evaluation; pharmaceutical products)

_____

3. 由于没有一种药物是完全安全的，消费者无法权衡潜在的益处和风险。(be in position to)

_____

4. 从广义上讲，国家监管部门的任务是保护和促进公众健康。(in broad terms)

_____

5. 对药品质量、安全性和疗效的判断应以科学为基础。(be based on)

_____

Listening & Speaking

Listening &
Speaking
Task 1

Task 1　Bob is in the emergency room at midnight. Listen to the conversation between Bob and the doctor and decide whether the following statements are true (T) or false (F).

Food Poisoning

( ) 1. Bob went to the hospital with a bad stomachache.

( ) 2. Bob had pain in the right lower stomach and upper abdomen, which spread to the head.

( ) 3. Bob didn't have diarrhea but kept vomiting.

( ) 4. Bob didn't feel so bad for the past few hours.

( ) 5. Most food borne illness symptoms present right away.

📖 **Notes**

1. Does the pain come and go or is it constant?
疼痛是时来时去还是持续不断？

2. It is constant, but sharpens at times, like a needle prick.

持续疼痛，但有时会变成锐痛，就像针刺一样。

3. food poisoning   食物中毒。

4. food borne illness   食源性疾病。

5. contaminated food   被污染的食物。

Task 2   Conrad Choiniere, Ph. D. , the director of the Office of Analytics and Outreach at FDA's Center for Food Safety and Applied Nutrition, is being interviewed by a reporter.

Listening &
Speaking
Task 2

What FDA Is Doing to Protect Consumers?

( ) 1. What contaminants are they talking about?

A. Bacteria in foods   B. Toxic metals in foods

C. Viruses in foods   D. Food additives

( ) 2. How do the contaminants get into our food supply?

A. Plants take environmental pollutants up as they grow

B. Plants are contaminated with pesticides

C. The food was contaminated during processing

D. There is man-made pollution in air, water and soil

( ) 3. Which of the following is not the work of the group?

A. Collecting data on food contamination

B. Collecting data on malnutrition

C. Studying the large amount data collected by FDA

D. Making a diet study

( ) 4. What group was the work aimed at?

A. The elderly   B. Children

C. Women   D. All of the above

( ) 5. What drives Dr. Conrad Choiniere to do this work?

A. To make money

B. To work with very dedicated people

C. To protect people and food we eat

D. To protect his family only

📖 Notes

1. Metals, such as arsenic, lead, cadmium, mercury and others are present in certain foods.

某些食物中存在金属，如砷、铅、镉、汞等。

2. We have been collecting data on contaminants and nutrients in foods for decades as part of our Total Diet Study.

几十年来，我们一直在收集食物中污染物和营养素的数据，作为我们总体饮食研究的一部分。

3. protect from   使免受，保护。

医药大学堂
WWW.YIYAODXT.COM

e. g. The body has natural defense mechanisms to protect it from disease.

人体对疾病具有先天性防御机制。

4. be concerned about　关心；挂念。

5. chronic health conditions　慢性疾病。

Task 3　Food safety is important in our life. Listen to the following passage and fill in the blanks with what you hear.

Keeping the family _____1_____ is a priority in any household. Being smart about how we shop for food can do a lot to help prevent exposure to the two most common food borne agents： _____2_____ and _____3_____. When it comes to food borne illness, most of us think of under-cooked meat and eggs. But the raw fruits and vegetables can pose a _____4_____, so can lunch, meat and deli-type salads. There are a few things you can do while at the grocery store： check the sell-by dates, use plastic bags for raw meat and poultry and keep them separated from the other groceries in your cart, and only buy pasteurized _____5_____ products and juice.

Task 4　Work in groups, try to discuss the topic of "Food Safety". Practice making the conversations with your partner according to what you hear in the Listening part.

Partner A	Partner B
Greet.	Greet and describe your physical condition.
Introduce the importance of food safety.	Ask the reason of food contamination.
Explain the reason.	Ask how to prevent food contamination.
Give effective preventive measures.	Ask Symptoms of food poisoning.
Explain how to deal with food poisoning.	Show the appreciation.

Reading B

National Medical Products Administration

What Is NMPA?

National Medical Products Administration （NMPA） is Chinese government's administrative body, which is responsible for regulating pharmaceuticals, medical devices, and cosmetics in China.

What Does NMPA Do?

NMPA is a vice-ministerial-level administrative agency under the State Administration for Market Regulation (SAMR). Specifically, NMPA is responsible for these 10 functions to regulate drugs, medical devices, and cosmetics in the Chinese mainland market:

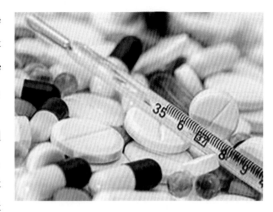

· Responsible for the safety supervision and management of drugs (including Chinese medicine, ethnic medicine, the same below), medical equipment and cosmetics. Formulate supervision and management policy planning, organize drafting of draft laws and regulations, formulate departmental regulations, and supervise implementation. Study and develop management and service policies that encourage new technologies and products for pharmaceuticals, medical devices, and cosmetics.

· Responsible for the standard management of pharmaceuticals, medical devices, and cosmetics. Organize the formulation and publication of national pharmacopeia and other pharmaceutical and medical device standards, organize the formulation of cosmetic standards, organize the development of a classification management system, and supervise the implementation. Participate in the formulation of the national essential medicines catalogs and cooperate with the implementation of the national essential medicine system.

· Responsible for the registration management of pharmaceuticals, medical devices and cosmetics. Formulate a registration management system, strictly review and approve the listing review, improve the facilitation measures for review and approval, and organize implementation.

· Responsible for the quality management of pharmaceuticals, medical devices, and cosmetics. Develop quality management practices and supervise implementation. Formulate production quality management regulations and implement them according to their duties. Develop management, use quality management practices and guide implementation.

· Responsible for risk management of drugs, medical devices, and cosmetics after listing. Organize the monitoring, evaluation, and disposal of adverse drug reactions, medical device adverse events and cosmetic adverse reactions. To undertake the safety emergency management of drugs, medical devices, and cosmetics in accordance with the law.

· Responsible for the admission management of licensed pharmacists. Formulate a system for the qualification of licensed pharmacists and guide the supervision of the registration of licensed pharmacists.

· Responsible for organizing and guiding the supervision and inspection of drugs, medical devices and cosmetics. Formulate an inspection system, investigate and deal with illegal acts in the registration of drugs, medical devices and cosmetics according to law, and organize and guide the investigation and punishment of illegal activities in production links.

· Responsible for foreign exchanges and cooperation in the field of supervision and management of pharmaceuticals, medical devices and cosmetics, and participate in the formulation of relevant international regulatory rules and standards.

· Responsible for guiding the work of drug supervision and administration departments of provinces, autonomous regions and municipalities directly under the Central Government.

· Completing other tasks assigned by the Party Central Committee and the State Council.

(465 words)

Words and Expressions			
device	/dɪˈvaɪs/	n.	装置；设备
cosmetic	/kɒzˈmetɪk/	n.	化妆品
ethnic	/ˈeθnɪk/	adj.	种族的；人种的
formulate	/ˈfɔːmjuleɪt/	vt.	规划
draft	/drɑːft/	vt.	起草；制定
participate	/pɑːˈtɪsɪpeɪt/	vi.	参与，参加；分享
catalog	/ˈkætəlɒg/	n.	目录
cooperate	/kəʊˈɒpəreɪt/	vi.	合作，配合；协力
monitor	/ˈmɒnɪtə (r) /	vt.	监控
disposal	/dɪˈspəʊzl/	n.	处理；支配
adverse	/ˈædvɜːs/	adj.	不利的；相反的
reaction	/rɪˈækʃn/	n.	反应，感应
accordance	/əˈkɔːdns/	n.	按照，依据；一致
illegal	/iˈliːgl/	adj.	非法的；违法的
relevant	/ˈreləvənt/	adj.	相关的；切题的
autonomous	/ɔːˈtɒnəməs/	adj.	自治的；自主的
municipality	/mjuːˌnɪsɪˈpæləti/	n.	市政当局；自治市或区
Proper Names			
National Medical Products Administration (NMPA)		国家药品监督管理局	
State Administration for Market Regulation (SAMR)		国家市场监督管理总局	
the Party Central Committee and the State Council		中国共产党中央委员会，简称中共中央	
the State Council		国务院	

After-reading Exercises

Task 1　Read the passage and choose the correct answer to each question.

(　　) 1. What is the NMPA not responsible for regulating? .

　　　　A. Drugs　　　　　　　　　　　B. Medical devices

　　　　C. Foods　　　　　　　　　　　D. Cosmetics

(　　) 2. Which of the following is not the main duty of NMPA?

　　　　A. It is responsible for creating policies, plans and standards governing the quality and safety of drugs, cosmetics, and medical devices

　　　　B. It is responsible for supervising the implementation of policies, plans and standards governing the quality and safety of drugs, cosmetics, and medical devices

　　　　C. It oversees standards-setting, registration, and quality management of drugs, cosmetics,

and medical devices

D. It oversees post-market inspection and risk management and registration of medical practitioner

(　　) 3. Which of the following is not included in the NMPA safety supervision of drugs?

A. Beverage　　　　　　　　　　B. Chinese medicine

C. Ethnic medicine　　　　　　　　D. Herb

(　　) 4. Which of the following does not belong to the registration management of pharmaceuticals, medical devices and cosmetics?

A. Formulating a registration management system

B. Strictly reviewing and approving the listing review

C. Improving the facilitation measures for review and approval

D. Organizing assessment

(　　) 5. What does risk management include except _____?

A. Organizing the monitoring, evaluation, and disposal of adverse drug reactions

B. Organizing the manufacture, evaluation, and disposal of medical devices

C. Organizing the monitoring, evaluation, and disposal of cosmetic adverse reactions

D. Undertaking the safety emergency management of drugs, medical devices, and cosmetics in accordance with the law

Task 2　Translate the following sentences into Chinese.

1. NMPA is Chinese government's administrative body, which is responsible for regulating pharmaceuticals, medical devices, and cosmetics in China.

_____

2. NMPA is responsible for the safety supervision and management of drugs (including Chinese medictne, ethnic medicine, the same below), medical equipment, and cosmetics.

_____

3. NMPA is responsible for the standard management of pharmaceuticals, medical devices, and cosmetics.

_____

4. NMPA organizes the monitoring, evaluation, and disposals of adverse drug reactions, medical device adverse events and cosmetic adverse reactions.

_____

5. NMPA formulates an inspection system, investigates and deals with illegal acts in the registration of drugs, medical devices and cosmetics according to law, and organizes and guides the investigation and punishment of illegal activities in production links.

_____

Practical Writing

Business Letters

英文商务信函是国际贸易业务往来的主要途径与方法。商务信函是重要的通讯工具，虽然电话、传真已被广泛应用，但仍需用书信做最后确认，且具有法律效力。特别是电子邮件普及后，通过电邮发送更为便捷。英文商务信函与普通书信的结构基本相同。

Sample

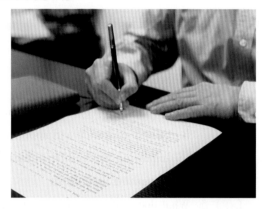

Inquiry

WESTIN CORPORATION

REGISTERED ADDRESS：20 WEST STREET，BROOKLYN NEW YORK 10268

PHONE：001-328-754-2389　FAX：(612) 918 2736　WEB SITE：WWW. WECO. COM

March 15，2020

Marketing Manager

Red East International Ltd.

18 South Street，Jing 'an District

Shanghai，200040

China

Dear Sir，

Will you please send us a copy of your catalogue and current pricelist for facemasks？We are interested in N95 respirator，surgical masks and basic cloth face mask.

We are the leading medical device dealers in New York，and have 23 branches in the country. If the quality of your product is satisfactory and the prices are reasonable，we would like to place regular orders for fairly large numbers with you.

Yours sincerely，

WESTIN CORPORATION

(Signature)

R. James

Sales Manager

商务信函通常包含以下项目：

信头（Letterhead）：商务信函基本采用事先印刷好信头的信纸。它的信头包括寄件人所在的单位名称、地址、邮政编码、电报、电传、电话号码等，通常居于信纸上方中间。

收件人姓名和地址（Inside Address）：这部分包括收件人姓名、头衔和地址等，一般在日期下方

1~2 行靠左书写。这部分的顺序是：收件人姓名、头衔（或职务、职称）、单位名称和地址。

称呼（The Salutation）：称呼在收件人地址下方 1~2 行书写，常用 Sir（s）。

正文（The Body of the Letter）：书信正文位于称呼下方 1~2 行书写。常用格式齐头式或缩进式。

结束语（The Complimentary Close）：位于书信正文两行，且与上方信头日期对齐。常用 Yours truly/Truly yours；Yours sincerely/Sincerely yours。

签名（The Signature）：在结尾处打印出大写的单位全称和写信人的全名，亲笔签名签在公司名称和打印姓名之间。

其他（The others）：有的书信还有附件（Enclosure）和附言（Postscript）。

Task   Write a business letter in English covering the following information.

寄件人姓名地址：中国上海静安区南街 18 号，东方红国际有限公司，市场部经理张林，邮编 200040，电话 86-021-62888888，传真 86－021－6288866。

收件人姓名地址：美国纽约布鲁克林区西街 20 号，威斯汀公司销售部经理 R. 詹姆斯，邮编 10268。发信日期：2020 年 3 月 20 日。

正文：

亲爱的詹姆斯先生：

谢谢贵公司 3 月 15 日来函，我们十分乐意与贵公司建立贸易关系。

我们将寄去你方所需的资料，并附上商品目录，以及我们出口货物的详细情况和价格。我相信我们公司的货物质量及价格是极其具有竞争性的。

等候贵方回复。

RED EAST INTERNATIONAL Ltd.
REGISTERED ADDRESS：18 SOUTH STREET, JING AN DISTRICT SHANGHAI, 200040
PHONE：_____   FAX：_____   WEBSITE：_____
_____
_____
Dear _____,
_____
_____
_____
_____
_____
_____

Grammar Tips

主谓一致，是指主语和谓语动词要保持人称、数、格、性等方面的一致。英语中动词 be 的变化形式最多，如 I am，You are，He is，We are。主语 I 一定要用 am 的动词形式，这就叫"主谓一致"。数的一致有如下三条基本原则：

Concord

Principle	Content
语法一致 grammatical concord	主语为单数形式，谓语动词也采取单数形式；主语为复数形式，谓语动词也采取复数形式（不包括复数形式单数概念的名词）
	e. g. Her child has no intention of spending a vacation with her. 她的孩子不想和她一起度假。 Her children have no intention of spending a vacation with her. 她的孩子们不想和她一起度假。
意义一致 notional concord	谓语动词的单、复数形式要取决于主语所表达的概念，而不取决于表面的语法标志 1. 主语形式虽为单数，但意义上却为复数，谓语动词用复数 2. 主语形式为复数，而意义上却是单数，谓语动词用单数
	e. g. The crowd were fighting for their lives. 人们在为他们的生命而战斗。 Three years in a strange land seems like a long time. 在一个陌生的地方呆三年似乎是一段很长的时间
就近一致 principle of proximity	谓语动词的单、复数形式取决于最靠近它的词语
	e. g. There is a square table and some chairs in the center of the dining-room. 餐厅中央有一张方桌和几把椅子。

Task 1　Please correct the underlined italics part in the following sentences.

1. The girl *show* her grandmother much attention.　　　　_____

2. A man of abilities *is* needed.　　　　_____

3. Ten minutes *are* enough.　　　　_____

4. Tom and his twin brother naturally *looks* a lot alike.　　　　_____

5. Here *are* a desk and a few chairs.　　　　_____

6. Neither of them *want* to go to the party.　　　　_____

7. Nobody but James and Jerry *were* there.　　　　_____

8. There *are* some paper, a pencil and three books on the desk.　　　　_____

9. The impossible *have* often proved possible.　　　　_____

10. Many a student *are* interested in this project.　　　　_____

Task 2　Choose the best answer to complete each sentence according to the principle of concord.

( ) 1. What he saw _____ two young men attacking the policeman.

A. was　　　　　　　　　　　　B. were

C. has　　　　　　　　　　　　D. has been

( ) 2. He as well as I _____ you.

A. agree with　　　　　　　　　B. agrees with

C. agree to　　　　　　　　　　D. agrees to

( ) 3. Neither Jane nor her parents _____ at home.

A. has　　　　　　　　　　　　B. is

C. are　　　　　　　　　　　　D. was

( ) 4. All that can be done _____ .

    A. has been done   B. have been done

    C. have done   D. has done

( ) 5. More than one _____ dismissed.

    A. are   B. is

    C. has been   D. have been

( ) 6. The young _____ the vital forces in modern society.

    A. is   B. are

    C. has been   D. have been

( ) 7. Mary is one of the girls who _____ always on time.

    A. has   B. was

    C. is   D. are

( ) 8. My classmate James and his friend _____ in the library.

    A. is   B. was

    C. are   D. are being

( ) 9. Trail and error _____ the source of our knowledge.

    A. are   B. is

    C. were   D. was

( ) 10. The majority of the students _____ .

    A. like music   B. likes music

    C. like the music   D. likes the music

Supplementary Reading

Public Medical Insurance and Universal Healthcare in China

What Is The Public Medical Insurance in China?

To achieve universal health coverage by 2020, China has implemented comprehensive reforms to improve medical insurance. China has three basic health insurance schemes: Urban Employee Basic Medical Insurance (UEBMI), Urban Resident Basic Medical Insurance (URBMI), and the New Rural Cooperative Medical System (NRCMS).

In China, urban employee basic medical insurance is obligatory insurance and the healthcare costs are paid by the employer and employee. Although the contributions to it vary from one municipality to another, they are usually 6% of the salary cost for the employer and 2% of the salary for the employee. The self-employed can also benefit from this insurance but must make all contributions.

For non-enterprise residents, health insurance is paid for by themselves and the state. For the unemployed or those on social assistance, insurance is subsidized by the state.

The New Rural Cooperative Medical Care System is proposed by the central government in China to finance farmers who face high medical costs for severe diseases or injuries. It is a multi-channel fundraising system composed by the government, collectives and individuals.

What Exactly Is Covered by Public Medical Insurance?

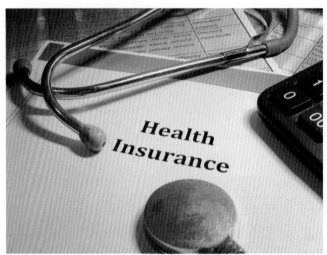

Publicly-financed basic medical insurance typically covers:

· inpatient hospital care

· primary and specialist care

· prescription drugs

· mental health care

· physical therapy

· emergency care

· Traditional Chinese Medicine

Cost-sharing, Co-payments and Reimbursements

Inpatient and outpatient care, including prescription drugs, are subject to different deductibles, co-payments, and reimbursement ceilings depending on the insurance plan, region, type of hospital (community, secondary, or tertiary), and other factors:

· Co-payments for outpatient physician visits are often small (5-10 Yuan), although physicians with professor titles have much higher co-payments.

· Prescription drug co-payments vary: in 2018 in Beijing, this was between 50% and 80% of the cost of the drug, depending on the hospital type.

· Co-payments for inpatient admissions are much higher than for outpatient services.

The public insurance programs only reimburse patients up to a certain ceiling, above which residents must cover all out-of-pocket costs. There are no annual caps on out-of-pocket spending. Reimbursement ceilings are significantly lower for outpatient care than for inpatient care. For example, in 2018, the outpatient care ceiling was 3,000 Yuan for Beijing residents with Urban Resident Basic Medical Insurance. In comparison, the ceiling for inpatient care was 200,000 Yuan. Annual deductibles have to be met before reimbursements, and different annual deductibles may apply for outpatient and inpatient care.

Preventive services, such as cancer screenings and flu vaccinations, are covered by a separate public health program. Children and the elderly have no co-payments for these services, but other residents have to pay 100% of these services out-of-pocket.

People can use out-of-network health services (even across provinces), but these have higher co-payments.

Safety Nets

For individuals who are not able to afford individual premiums for publicly-financed health insurance, or cannot cover out-of-pocket spending, a medical financial assistance program——funded by local governments and social donations——serves as a safety net in both urban and rural.

How Is Healthcare Provided?

Primary care is delivered primarily by:

· Village doctors and community health workers in rural clinics.

· General practitioners (GPs) or family doctors in rural township and urban community hospitals.

· Medical professionals (doctors and nurses) in secondary and tertiary hospitals.

(549 words)

After-reading Exercises

Task　Decide whether the following statements are true (T) or false (F) according to the text.

(　　) 1. In China, Urban Employee Basic Medical Insurance is obligatory insurance and all the healthcare costs are paid by the employer.

(　　) 2. The self-employed can't benefit from the public insurance if they don't make any contributions.

(　　) 3. Publicly-financed basic medical insurance covers Traditional Chinese Medicine.

(　　) 4. Co-payments for outpatient admissions are much higher than for inpatient services.

(　　) 5. For individuals who are not able to afford individual premiums for publicly-financed health insurance can get donations from local governments and society.

Vocabulary Tips

Root "-cosm-, -cosmo-"：世界，宇宙，装饰。

Example：cosmos 宇宙；macrocosm 宏观世界；cosmonautic 宇宙航行学；cosmopolitanism 世界主义；cosmetic 化妆品。

Prefix "dis- (di-, dif-)"：否定，相反；除去；分离，分开，散开；恶化；加强意义。dis-主要出现在c、p、r、s、t等字母前面；而di-则出现在l、m、r、v等字母前面，出现在v前面最为常见，dis-也成为一个活性词缀，能与英语中的单词相缀合，表示否定的意思；dif-出现在字母f前。

Example：disabled 残疾的；dispassionate 平心静气的；disposal 处理，支配；disseminate 散布，

传播;discriminate 辨别，歧视;disforest 砍伐森林;dissect 切开;divorce 离婚;differential 差别的，特异的。

Task Complete the sentences with the given words.

dissect	dispassionate	discriminate	cosmetic	macrocosm

1. The _____ of the universe is mirrored in the microcosm of the mind.

2. It is illegal to _____ on grounds of race, sex or religion.

3. It is true that science is empirical and _____ .

4. The definition of "_____" is to cut a plant or dead animal into separate parts for scientific examination.

5. The _____ brand is her favorite.

Proverbs and Sayings

◇An apple a day keeps the doctor away.

一天吃一个苹果有益于身体健康。

◇Feed by measure and defy physician.

饮食有节制，医生无用处。

◇Temperance and industry are the two real physicians of mankind.

节制与勤劳是人类两个真正的医生。

题库

Unit 10

The Future of Medicine

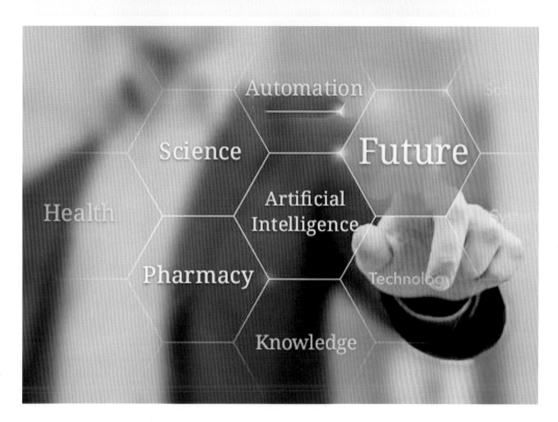

Unit Objectives

After studying this unit, you are expected to:

· master the vocabulary and technical terms related to the future of medicine;

· understand the future of medicine in China and Chinese medicine cuisine;

· know English punctuations correctly.

And you should learn how to:

· communicate with others about the symptoms and prevention measures of COVID-19 and pharmacy automation;

· write an abstract.

Introduction

The future of medicine has been an ongoing discussion for some years. The advances in technology of

Introduction

all kinds, and their impact on the profession, are a serious concern. With advances in artificial intelligence and 'fuzzy' logic (an approach to computing based on 'degrees of truth'), and in logistics and supply (e. g. advances in the design, and use of drones), we must be concerned for the future of medicine.

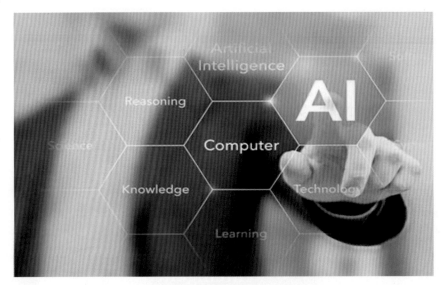

New technologies and treatments——precision medicine, digital therapeutics, 3D printing, immunotherapy, gene and stem cell therapies and artificial intelligence——have arrived or are on their way.

Warming-up

Task Work in groups. Match the pictures to the proper statements. Then check your answers with your partner.

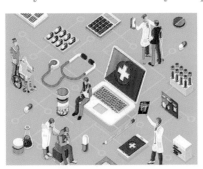

A

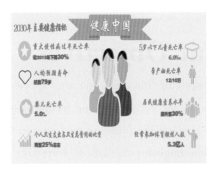

B

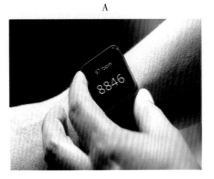

C

D

（　）1. The Chinese government's overarching idea is "big health", aiming to deliver a full suite of health services that cover the entire care continuum, with an emphasis on health management and chronic disease management.

（　）2. The use of smart devices and wearables that continuously collect health and contextual data, allowing patient monitoring anywhere.

（　）3. The willingness to engage with connected-care technology will have an important role to play in creating more and better access to healthcare solutions across the whole continuum of health.

（　）4. There is significant potential for digital transformation in the health sector.

Reading A

Reading A

"Big Health" and the Future of Medicine in China

The so-called Fourth Industrial Revolution is in full swing, bringing with it both disruption and opportunity. In healthcare specifically, digital transformation is impacting broadly and deeply, disrupting business models, services, regulations, and skills supply and demand.

The Chinese Healthcare Vacuum

The Chinese government's overarching idea is to move from "disease-centered" care to "big health", aiming to deliver a full suite of health services that cover the entire care continuum, with an emphasis on health management and chronic disease management. Chinese people and healthcare professionals alike recognize the importance of prevention in healthcare.

Overburdened Infrastructure

The pressures on an overburdened infrastructure have encouraged the Chinese government to embrace the role of technology in relieving the burden on an over-stretched healthcare system. Central to this is encouraging the application of big data to enable precise diagnosis and personalized healthcare. By 2020, three digital national databases will be established, incorporating health information, health profiles and medical records.

The scope of smart devices and wearables is significant, potentially leading to fewer readmissions, more rapid emergency responses, and more immediate care to avoid deterioration or adverse events, such as stroke or falls.

Building up cloud-based regional imaging centers to support low-tiered hospitals to ensure right-first-time diagnosis, and connecting

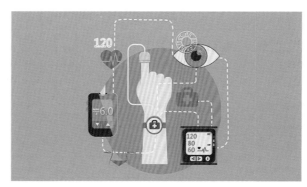

different levels of hospitals to enable data-sharing, remote consulting and two-way referral are just some of the ways in which digital technology will play a crucial role.

Embracing Connected Care

A large majority (92%) of Chinese healthcare professionals believe it is important that the healthcare system in China is integrated. And fortunately, the government has little to do to convince the general public about the benefits of health-related technology: they're already open to its applications and, in many cases, already using connected-care technology to track their own health.

The willingness to engage with connected-care technology will have an important role to play in creating more and better access to healthcare solutions across the whole continuum of health——from prevention to diagnosis, treatment to post-acute care.

A Digital Shift

There is significant potential for digital transformation in the sector——both in terms of creating efficiencies, but also harnessing new opportunities to improve patient outcomes. From advances in connected home and virtual care, to data-driven solutions that allow patient health to be monitored more effectively in real time, digital solutions are instrumental in accelerating the shift to value-based healthcare.

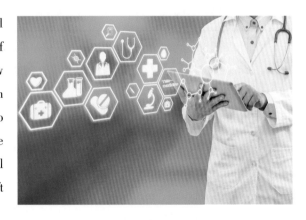

There are particularly significant gains to be made in prevention and home care. The move from primarily "inpatient" to "outpatient" settings will not only broaden geographic and demographic access, but will also signal a significant shift in the current healthcare model, freeing up resources.

While there is no denying certain existing structural and cultural barriers that need to be overcome——from reimbursement models and financial incentives to regulation, or even some basic concerns around trust——the Chinese government has shown significant commitment to embracing this shift. And, as pockets of activity are already proving, wider adoption of smart, connected technologies will continue to boost affordability and access.

(535 words)

Words and Expressions			
disruption	/dis'rʌpʃn/	n.	打乱，扰乱
overarching	/ˌəʊvər'ɑːtʃiŋ/	adj.	总体的；首要的
suite	/'swiːt/	n.	（一套）套间
continuum	/kən'tinjuəm/	n.	连续体
management	/'mænidʒmənt/	n.	管理
recognize	/'rekəgnaiz/	v.	认出；承认
overburdened	/ˌəʊvə'bɜːdənd/	adj.	负担过重的
infrastructure	/'infrəstrʌktʃə(r)/	n.	基础设施

Reading A
Words and
Expressions

医药大学堂
WWW.YIYAODXT.COM

续表

embrace	/im'breis/	vt.	拥抱；围绕
stretched	/'stretʃt/	adj.	拉伸的；延伸的
precise	/pri'sais/	adj.	精确的；明确的
incorporate	/in'kɔːpəreit/	vt.	包含；把……合并
scope	/'skəup/	n.	范围
wearable	/'weərəbl/	n.	可穿戴设备
readmission	/ˌriːəd'miʃn/	n.	再入院
deterioration	/diˌtiəriə'reiʃn/	n.	恶化
stroke	/strəuk/	n.	中风
tier	/tiə (r) /	n.	等级；层
remote	/ri'məut/	adj.	遥远的；远程的
referral	/ri'fɜːrəl/	n.	转诊
crucial	/kruː'ʃl/	adj.	重要的；决定性的
acute	/ə'kjuːt/	adj.	严重的；急性的
harness	/'hɑːnis /	vt.	利用
virtual	/'vɜːtʃuəl/	adj.	虚拟的
reimbursement	/ˌriːim'bɜːsmənt/	n.	报销；偿还
incentive	/in'sentiv/	n.	动机；刺激
commitment	/kə'mitmənt/	n.	承诺；保证
Proper Names			
The Fourth Industrial Revolution		第四次工业革命	

📖 Notes

1. The so-called Fourth Industrial Revolution is in full swing, bringing with it both disruption and opportunity.

所谓的第四次工业革命正在如火如荼地进行着，带来了颠覆和机遇。

"it" 指 "The so-called Fourth Industrial Revolution".

"bringing" 为现在分词作伴随状语，伴随状语的主语与主句的主语相同，都是"the so-called Fourth Industrial Revolution"；且"bringing with it…opportunity"这个动作与主句中的"is in full swing"这个状态为同时发生的。

本文中相同的用法还有"… disrupting business models, services, regulations, and skills and supply demand."

2. The Chinese government's overarching idea is to move from "disease-centered" care to "big health"…

中国政府的总体理念是从"以疾病为中心"的医疗转向"大健康"……

"disease-centered"，意为"以疾病为中心的"；为"名词 + 动词的过去分词"构成的形容词。

e.g. "cloud-based" 基于云的；"health-related" 与健康相关的；"value-based" 基于价值的。

3. And fortunately, …, in many cases, …their own health.

幸运的是，政府几乎没有做什么来说服公众相信健康相关技术的好处：他们已经接受健康相关的应用，而且在很多情况下，已经在使用互联医疗技术来追踪他们自己的健康状况。

"fortunately"副词作插入语;"in many cases"介词短语作插入语。

插入语指插在句子中的词语或句子,其位置比较灵活,通常被逗号、破折号或句子的其他部分隔开,与句中其他部分没有语法上的联系。

After-reading Exercises

Task 1　Answer the following questions according to the text.

1. In which aspect does digital transformation impact healthcare field?

_____

2. What is the overarching idea of the Chinese government?

_____

3. What will be incorporated within the three digital national databases?

_____

4. Why does the Chinese government have little to do to convince the general public about the benefits of health-related technology?

_____

5. What will be boosted with wider adoption of smart, connected technologies?

_____

Task 2　Match the words (1-10) to the Chinese meanings (a-j).

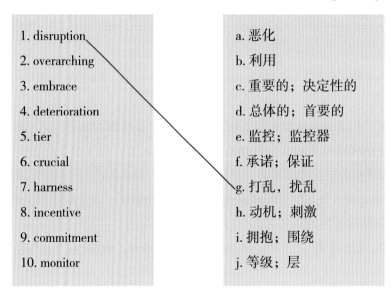

1. disruption
2. overarching
3. embrace
4. deterioration
5. tier
6. crucial
7. harness
8. incentive
9. commitment
10. monitor

a. 恶化
b. 利用
c. 重要的;决定性的
d. 总体的;首要的
e. 监控;监控器
f. 承诺;保证
g. 打乱,扰乱
h. 动机;刺激
i. 拥抱;围绕
j. 等级;层

Task 3　Fill in each blank with the proper form of the word or phrase given in brackets.

1. The _____ of Chinese Navy began decades ago. (transform)
2. I told you the story to _____ the devotion of doctors. (emphasis)
3. They fear that the situation might _____ into full-scale war. (deteriorate)
4. He has called for an _____ of political reforms. (accelerate)
5. The _____ only seemed to make the thing worse. (deny)

Task 4   Translate the following sentences into English using the words or phrases you have learned in this unit.

1. 所谓的第四次工业革命正在如火如荼地进行着，带来了颠覆和机遇。（bring with）

_____

2. 中国民众和卫生保健专业人员都认识到预防在卫生保健中的重要性。（recognize）

_____

3. 政府几乎没有做什么来说服公众相信健康相关技术的好处。（convince）

_____

4. 他们已经在使用连接医疗技术来追踪自己的健康状况。（track）

_____

5. 智能、互联技术的广泛应用将继续提高人们看得起病的能力和增加看病的途径。（boost）

_____

Listening & Speaking

Task 1   Daniela and Elizabeth are talking about the symptoms of COVID-19. Listen to the conversation and decide whether the following statements are true (T) or false (F).

Listening & Speaking Task 1

What are the Symptoms of COVID-19?

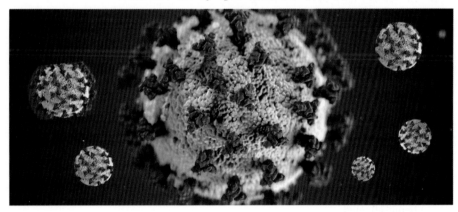

( ) 1. There are a range of symptoms from mild to severe.

( ) 2. Every patient develops symptoms.

( ) 3. Common symptoms include fever, fatigue and some respiratory symptoms.

( ) 4. Some patients become blind and deaf after being affected.

( ) 5. Severe cases may report pneumonia or organ failure.

📖 **Notes**

1. a range of   一系列，很多。

2. fatigue n. 疲劳，疲乏。

3. sore adj. 疼痛的，酸痛的。

Listening & Speaking Task 2

4. rash n. 皮疹。

Task 2 COVID-19 spreads everywhere. Daniela and Elizabeth are talking about the way to prevent transmission. Listen to the conversation and choose the best answer to each question you hear.

How to Prevent Transmission of COVID-19?

( ) 1. What can people do to prevent transmission?
  A. Wear a mask
  B. Wash hands regularly with soap and running water
  C. Both A and B
  D. Not mentioned

( ) 2. How far should people keep with others?
  A. People doesn't have to keep distant from others
  B. For at least 1 meter
  C. For at least 2 meters
  D. As far as possible

( ) 3. What should people do when he is coughing or sneezing?
  A. Cover his mouth with his hands
  B. Cover his nose with his hands
  C. Cover his mouth and nose with a flexed elbow
  D. He doesn't have to do anything

( ) 4. What should people do if he doesn't feel well?
  A. Go to the hospital directly
  B. Take medicine without any medical consultation
  C. Stay home and call a hotline
  D. He doesn't have to do anything

( ) 5. Decide the following statements, which one is wrong?
  A. Stay home if people are feeling unwell and call a hotline
  B. Wear a mask, wash hands regularly and keep at least 1 meter with others to prevent being affected
  C. If people have a fever, cough or difficulty breathing, seek medical care early
  D. Don't tell the healthcare provider anything

Notes

1. transmission n. 传播。
2. prevent … from … 阻止，防止。
3. hand rub 速干手消毒剂。

Listening & Speaking Task 3

Task 3 An antibody test detects antibodies to the virus. Listen to the following passage and fill in the blanks with what you hear.

If an antibody test finds antibodies in the blood, it likely means the person has been _____ 1 infected with the virus. Antibody tests do not show if you have a ____2____ infection and should not be used to diagnose a current infection from COVID-19.

The results from antibody tests can help us better understand questions about ____3____ to COVID-19 by helping identify: who has been infected and has developed antibodies; if antibodies may provide protection from future infection; who may still be at risk; or who may be ____4____ to donate a part of their blood called convalescent plasma, which may serve as a possible ____5____ for those who are seriously ill from COVID-19.

Task 4　Work in groups, try to discuss the topic of "What are the symptoms of COVID-19?" and "How to prevent transmission of COVID-19?" Practice making the conversations with your partner according to what you hear in the Listening part.

Partner A	Partner B
Greet.	Greet and ask the pandemic.
Tell the seriousness.	Ask the symptoms of COVID–19.
Express the common symptoms and the symptoms of severe cases.	Ask the effective ways to prevent transmission.
Explain the effective ways of preventing.	What should people do when feeling unwell?
Stay home and seek medical care.	Show the appreciation.

Reading B

Pharmacy Automation

Pharmacy automation involves the automation of everyday pharmacy tasks. For example, the dispensing of medication, data handling and traditional management of prescriptions.

With rapid technological advancement in the field of automation and robotics, researchers are striving to provide a wide range of solutions for pharmacy management. These automated solutions range from basic dispensing and packaging of medications to more complex and advanced tasks such as handling of inventory and financial management.

Benefits of Pharmacy Automation

The integration of automation and robotics in the field of pharmacy has significantly improved security, storage, and labelling features. Due to the amazing benefits offered by AI and automation, even traditional setups have started to make the switch.

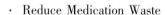

· Improved Efficiency

Automation surpasses the expertise and knowledge of the most attentive and professional pharmacists. Especially when it comes to accuracy and speed, machines can definitely be the safest bid. Apart from that, pharmacy automation has also improved the productivity factor by elevating the total number of prescriptions filled, which noticeably is far greater than what pharmacists used to achieve with manual working.

· Reduce Medication Waste

Pharmacists using the best automation practices can also control the potential medication waste that can occur from the filling or labelling processes.

· Better Counseling

Pharmacy automation has been closely linked with reducing the amount of manual workload on pharmacists. As a result, the pharmacy staff can better counsel patients and answer their queries.

· Reduced Labor Costs

Did you know the average pharmacist walks around 8 miles each day in a pharmacy doing various pharmacy tasks? Pharmacy automation enables pharmacists to automate ongoing pharmacy tasks, including filling prescriptions, labelling, and dispensing. Automation in pharmacy ensures reduced labour costs and also helps alleviate stress in the working environment.

· Ensure Safety

The chances of human error in the pharmacy sector can be particularly dangerous when pharmacists are dispensing strictly regulated medications and drugs. For example, a pharmacy worker can provide confidential information in a voicemail, which can risk the safety or confidentiality of the company or the patient.

Pharmacies can significantly reduce such types of risks by integrating automated calling programs designed to provide only instructed information to the patients.

Pharmacy Automation Trends

· Counting Scale

Counting scales are small-sized devices that can fit in any pharmacy space. These counters come with a barcode scanner to scan the label and the prescription bottle.

· Tablet Counting Device

Tablet counting tools are equipped with scanners and information screens. These devices allow you to examine the label and scan the bottle to confirm that you're dispensing the right medicine.

In addition to that, you can also integrate your tablet counting tool with your pharmacy management system to streamline your workflow and reduce the risk of errors.

· Dispensing and Packaging Robots

Dispensing and packaging robots perform different tasks based on your requirements. Some dispensing robots are used to read the prescription and select and dispense the right medication from the storage. Similarly, some robots can store vials and labels.

Packaging robots, on the other hand, are used to pack pills and medications in a smart way so that your patients don't need a pill organizer to take their routine medicines.

Pharmacy automation has transformed the way traditional community pharmacies used to work earlier. With pharmacy automation, pharmacies can streamline their workflow and achieve better efficiency.

(548 words)

Words and Expressions

robotics	/rəʊˈbɒtiks/	n.	机器人技术
integration	/ˌintiˈgreiʃn/	n.	整合，集成
surpass	/səˈpɑːs/	vt.	超越
attentive	/əˈtentiv/	adj.	专心的
bid	/bid/	n.	出价
manual	/ˈmænjuəl/	adj.	手控的；用手的
sector	/ˈsektə/	n.	部门
confidential	/ˌkɒnfiˈdenʃl/	adj.	机密的
barcode	/ˈbɑːkəʊd/	n.	条形码
scanner	/ˈskænə/	n.	扫描仪
streamline	/ˈstriːmlain/	vt.	组织；集成
vial	/ˈvaiəl/	n.	小瓶；药水瓶
routine	/ruːˈtiːn/	adj.	常规的，例行的
transform	/ˈtrænsˈfɔːm/	vt.	改变；转换

Proper Names

Pharmacy Automation	药房自动化
AI (artificial intelligence)	人工智能

After-reading Exercises

Task 1   Read the passage and choose the correct answer to each question.

(   ) 1. Everyday pharmacy tasks include _____ .

A. the dispensing of medication

B. data handling

  C. traditional management of prescription

  D. All of the above

( ) 2. Which of the following is not the benefit of pharmacy automation?

  A. Less financial cost

  B. Improved efficiency

  C. Reduced medication waste and labor costs

  D. Better counseling

( ) 3. With the help of pharmacy automation, pharmacists may achieve all of the following, except

  _____ .

  A. better counseling patients

  B. increasing work stress

  C. better answering patients' queries

  D. walking less within the pharmacy

( ) 4. Pharmacy automation trends include _____ .

  A. counting scale

  B. tablet counting device

  C. dispensing and packaging robots

  D. All of the above

( ) 5. According to the passage, which of the following is wrong?

  A. Pharmacy automation surpasses pharmacists in every aspect

  B. Automated calling program provides only instructed information

  C. Counting scales fit only spacious pharmacy

  D. Dispensing and packaging robots perform on requirements

Task 2 Translate the following sentences into Chinese.

1. The integration of automation and robotics in the field of pharmacy has significantly improved security, storage, and labelling features.

_____

2. Automation surpasses the expertise and knowledge of the most attentive and professional pharmacists.

_____

3. Pharmacists can significantly reduce such types of risks by integrating automated calling programs designated to provide only instructed information to the patients.

_____

4. Dispensing and packaging robots perform different tasks based on your requirements.

_____

5. Pharmacy automation has transformed the way traditional community pharmacies used to work earlier.

_____

Practical Writing

Abstract

摘要以提供文献内容梗概为目的，不加评论和补充解释，简明、确切地记述文献重要内容的短文。

摘要是学术论文的重要组成部分，应同时包含中文摘要及英文摘要。摘要应具有独立性和自明性，并且拥有与文献同等量的主要信息，即不阅读全文就能获得必要的信息。

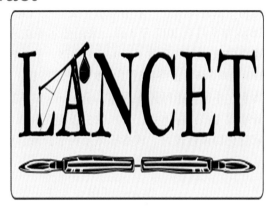

摘要通常包含以下 4 个部分：

目的（Objective）：阐述研究的目的、范围、重要性。

方法（Method）：采用什么手段和方法等进行研究。

结果（Results）：阐述通过研究获得的定性、定量的试验数据和结果。

结论（Conclusion）：对研究结果进行分析研究的基础上得出的结论性判断、评价和建议等。

Sample

**Development of a Performance Appraisal System for Essential
Public Health Service Delivery Institutions in Chongqing**

〔Abstract〕Objective   To develop a performance appraisal system for essential public health service delivery institutions in Chongqing, providing an objective reference for evaluating the performance of institutions in Chongqing and other regions of western China in implementing public health programs. Methods   We developed the initial Performance Appraisal System for Essential Public Health Service Delivery Institutions in Chongqing (PASEPHSDIC) and Expert Consultation Questionnaire based on the relative policies in Chongqing and China, literature review and other methods as well as the PASEPHSDIC (2016 edition). Using Delphi method, we determined the indicators and corresponding weight coefficients of the final version of PASEPHSDIC. Results   From September 2016 to March 2017, we conducted 2 rounds of Delphi expert consultation, and both of them achieved a 100.0% response rate. The overall authority coefficient (Cr) was 0.878. The Kendall's W for the first and second round of consultation was 0.320 and 0.386, respectively. The final version of PASEPHSDIC consists of 5 first-level indicators, 26 second-level indicators and 67 third-level indicators, with weight assigned to each indicator. The Cronbach's α for the whole system was 0.666. Conclusion   The PASEPHSDIC was developed with high response rate, authority degree and good consensus from experts, although the Kendall's W of the second round of consultation was higher than that of the first round. This system is scientific and reasonable, which can be used as a tool for objectively assessing the quality of essential public health services in Chongqing.

重庆市基本公共卫生服务绩效考核指标体系构建研究

【摘要】目的　构建重庆市基本公共卫生服务绩效考核指标体系，为重庆市及西部各地区公共卫生服务项目绩效评估提供客观参考。方法　结合我国和重庆市相关政策，采用文献分析等研究方法，以2016年重庆市基本公共卫生服务项目绩效评估指标体系为基础，初步建立绩效考核评估体系并编制专家咨询问卷。采用德尔菲法，经两轮专家咨询，确定绩效考核指标及其权重系数。结果　于2016年9月至2017年3月，采用德尔菲法进行专家咨询。两轮专家咨询表的回收率均为100.0%。专家总体权威程度系数（Cr）为0.878。第1轮和第2轮专家咨询的指标总体协调系数（W）分别为0.320和0.386。最终构建了由5项一级指标、26项二级指标、67项三级指标及其权重构成的评价指标体系。本研究指标体系总体Cronbach's α系数为0.666。结论　本研究构建了重庆市基本公共卫生服务绩效考核指标体系，专家的积极程度和权威程度均较高，第2轮专家意见协调程度优于第1轮，专家意见协调性较好。该指标体系科学合理，能客观评估重庆市基本公共卫生服务水平。

Task

2015—2018年重庆市毕业后全科医生教育开展情况研究

【摘要】目的　深入分析2015—2018年重庆市毕业后全科医生教育开展情况，查找问题所在，提出建议。方法　收集重庆市55家全科培训基地2015—2018年全科医师规范化培训、助理全科医生培训参培人员年龄、学历、身份、持证情况、工作岗位等信息，分析培养规模和参培情况。结果　2015—2018年全科医师规范化培训，参培人员的学历以本科为主，占总人数的92.53%，2018年本科生为95.24%，较2015年的89.42%增加5.82%；参培人员应以应届毕业生和单位人为主，应届生占总人数的60%~70%，以农村订单定向培养学员为主，占80%左右。2016—2018年助理全科医生培训，参培人员的学历以专科为主，占总人数的98.99%；参培人员中，应届毕业生占总人数的58.67%。结论　目前重庆市毕业后全科医生教育存在助理全科医生培训启动晚且规模不足的问题；下一步应继续坚持开展临床医学专业（本科）农村订单定向医学生免费培养，沿用属地化免费医学专科生培训，同时尽快启动专科层次农村订单定向医学生免费培养，并适度扩大助理全科医生培训规模。

The Situation of General Practitioner Education after Graduation in Chongqing from 2015 to 2018

[Abstract] Objective _____, this paper tries to find out the existing problems and put forward some suggestions. Methods　Of GPs and assistant GPs _____ in Chongqing were collected. And the training scale and situation were analyzed. Results　From 2015 to 2018, was mainly undergraduate, accounting for 92.53% of the total number. In 2018, the number of undergraduateswas 95.24%, an increase of 5.82% compared with 89.42% in 2015. The participants were mainly _____, accounting for 60%-70% of the total number of fresh students, and mainly rural _____, accounting for about 80%. In 2016-2018, the training of assistant general practitioners was mainly based on _____, accounting for 98.99% of the total number; among the participants, _____ accounted for 58.67% of the total number. Conclusion　At present, the training of assistant GPs starts late and _____. In the next step, we should _____ for rural order – oriented students (undergraduates) of _____. At the same time, _____ should be started as soon as possible, and the training scale of assistant GPs should be _____.

Grammar Tips

在英语书面语中，标点符号发挥着分隔作用，并拥有指明语法关系和语义的功能。
下面大家来学习一下英语书面语中，最常见的9种标点符号的作用和用法。

Punctuations

标点	符号	用法
逗号 Comma	,	用于分隔并列成分、分句、同位语、状语、非限制性定语从句、直接引语和导语
		e. g. Honestly, Mrs. Li, the English teacher, loves her students, and her students love her too.
句号 Full Stop	.	用于陈述句、语气温和的祈使句之后；用于某些缩略词之后
		e. g. Prof. Wang is giving a lecture at present.
问号 Question Mark	?	用于疑问句、委婉的祈使句之后
		e. g. It is cold outside, isn't it? Please open the window, would you?
冒号 Colon	:	用于引出表示列举、解释或说明性的词语 引出对前文进行总结、补充的词语
		e. g. The arrangement of semi-final matches are as follows: Brazil VS China, USA VS Russia.
分号 Semicolon	;	用于分隔地位平等的独立子句
		e. g. On the committee are quite a few well-knownexperts; for example, Mr. Zhao, editor-in-chief of the local newspaper; Professor Xu, Dean of the Institute; and Miss He, President of the General Hospital.
感叹号 Exclamation Point	!	用于感叹句，表示感叹、赞美、嘲讽等 用于祈使句，表示命令或强烈情感
		e. g. Merry Christmas! Be quiet!
引号 Quotation Mark	" "	用于引出直接引语；引述书名、文章名称、电影名称等
		e. g. "Why didn't you come to the party last night?" "The Sound of Music" is a very moving film.
连字符 Hyphen	-	用于连接复合词、数字中的十位数和个位数，连接词缀与词根
		e. g. The world-famous scientist is sixty-seven years old.
省字号 Apostrophe	'	构成名词所有格或简略形式
		e. g. Max's dictionary is on the desk, isn't it?

**Task 1   Mark the sentence(s) with correct punctuation with tick √ (Correct).
Then make necessary corrections in all the other sentence(s).**

1. Helen Keller was born on June 27th 1880.   _____

2. Do you hear me.   _____

3. For example Lily and Lucy are twins.   _____

4. When you read classic English works, you will often find names like Jane, Elizabeth, Mary and Dori.

   _____

5. These are the things I want in life, a spacious apartment, a loving wife and a smart child.

   _____

6. Henry's son will be the next King. _____

7. Sally said, Yes, I do. _____

8. Happy New Year! _____

9. The kind hearted lady is popular among the community. _____

10. Lisa is on the left; Amber is on the right. _____

Task 2   Choose the best punctuation to complete each sentence.

(　　) 1. Look out _____

      A. !　　　　　　　　　　　　　B. .

      C. ;　　　　　　　　　　　　　D. ,

(　　) 2. He is tall _____ strong and handsome.

      A. :　　　　　　　　　　　　　B. ;

      C. -　　　　　　　　　　　　　D. ,

(　　) 3. "The most popular teacher of this year" goes to Prof _____ Kevau.

      A. ,　　　　　　　　　　　　　B. .

      C. '　　　　　　　　　　　　　D. "

(　　) 4. This is a two _____ way road.

      A. '　　　　　　　　　　　　　B. :

      C. -　　　　　　　　　　　　　D. "

(　　) 5. I sawJoy _____ s football on the ground.

      A. -　　　　　　　　　　　　　B. :

      C. '　　　　　　　　　　　　　D. ,

(　　) 6. Please close the door, will you _____

      A. .　　　　　　　　　　　　　B. ?

      C. !　　　　　　　　　　　　　D. -

(　　) 7. The names of the students who get grade A in the exam are as follows _____ Jerry, Michael, Max and Bruce.

      A. ,　　　　　　　　　　　　　B. -

      C. ;　　　　　　　　　　　　　D. :

(　　) 8. Nicola was watching basketball on TV _____ he was doing his homework as well.

      A. ;　　　　　　　　　　　　　B. ,

      C. :　　　　　　　　　　　　　D. -

(　　) 9. Matt says _____ "My son and I are going to help them. "

      A. ,　　　　　　　　　　　　　B. .

      C. ;　　　　　　　　　　　　　D. :

(　　) 10. However _____ be prepared to listen carefully.

      A. ,　　　　　　　　　　　　　B. '

      C. ;　　　　　　　　　　　　　D. :

Supplementary Reading

Chinese Medicinal Cuisine

A lot of people all over the world like to eat Chinese food, but Chinese medicinal cuisine is a special type——an ancient healing art you can explore. It is a kind of traditional Chinese medicine.

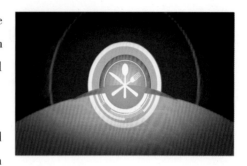

A Brief History of Medicinal Cuisine

Authentic Chinese medicinal food dishes are prepared according to traditional recipes and techniques, based on ancient ideas about how the human body operates. They described the effect of each kind of meat, grain, herb, or vegetable on the human body, how the body operates, and gave suggestions about what to prepare to stay healthy or cure disease.

The earliest work is *The Yellow Emperor's Classic of Internal Medicine*, which contains the basic ideas of Chinese food therapy. It gave recommendations on what to eat for different health conditions and different environmental conditions.

Ancient Chinese medical books list hundreds of plant, animal, and chemical ingredients and tell their specific effects on the human body. These books give ideas about the physical principles involved in human health, and they describe how herbs or special foods help, along with TCM techniques such as moxibustion and acupuncture.

The General Principles of Chinese Medicinal Cuisine

· Balance

The basic idea is to balance the qi and the body fluids——the fundamentals of Chinese traditional medicine. It is thought that a healthy body or organ has a proper balance of these things. When they are out of balance, there is disease or sickness.

The environment or physical injury disrupts the balance. For example, cold weather causes a lack of qi or high yin in the body. So high yang foods are eaten. In hot weather when there is naturally too much yang, high yin foods are eaten.

· Adding Medicinal Herbs

Healing herbs or animal parts can be added to the diet to heal disease. Many of the same herbs are used by Western herbalists and herbalists in other parts of the world for the same conditions, so this strongly suggests that the herbs have real medicinal effects.

· Using Heats and Flavors

All foods are categorized by qi temperature, ranging from high yang to high yin, and one of the five food flavors (sour, sweet, bitter, hot and salty). A food item's qi temperature and specific flavor influences the body in its own way.

It is thought that people should generally include all the flavors in every meal and balance the "heat". Most Chinese people think that if too much of one type of food is consumed, it can cause an imbalance in the body.

· Mealtime TCM Principles

The ancient texts described not only what to prepare for meals, but also how to eat meals. You might be surprised at these Chinese customs about eating meals that have been part of the culture for hundreds of years.

· Try to avoid overly processed food. Eat naturally.

· Eat seasonal vegetables and fruits.

· Always make sure the vegetables are cooked.

· Sit down to eat at a quiet place.

· Chew the food well.

· Eat slowly.

· Pay attention to your eating, and get away from distractions. In TCM your mind plays a part in how well you digest food, so pay attention to the tastes of the food.

· Do not skip meals.

· After lunch, take a nap or rest for a while.

(443 words)

After-reading Exercises

Task　Decide whether the following statements are true (T) or false (F) according to the text.

(　　) 1. Chinese medicinal cuisine is a special type of Chinese food.

(　　) 2. The basic ideas about food and health have changed a lot.

(　　) 3. To keep balance, yang foods are eaten in cold weather; and yin foods are eaten in hot weather.

(　　) 4. Healing herbs or animal parts can be added to the diet to heal disease.

(　　) 5. According to TCM principles, if a person doesn't want to have dinner, he may skip it.

Vocabulary Tips

Root "immuno- "：免疫。

Example：immunotherapy 免疫疗法；immunoglobulin 免疫球蛋白，免疫血球素；immunology 免疫学；immunohistochemistry 免疫组织化学。

Root "-stru-, -struct-"：建设，结构。

Example：construction 建造，建筑物；infrastructure 基础设施；destruction 毁灭，破坏；obstruction 阻碍，障碍物；instruct 指示，教育。

Task   Complete the sentences with the given words.

| immunoglobulin | immunotherapy | instruction | construct | self-destruct |

1. _____ is the prevention or treatment of disease with substances that stimulate the immune response.

2. They're going to be famous, but unless something happens, they're going to _____ .

3. _____ is any of a class of proteins present in the serum (血清；免疫血清) and cells of the immune system, which function as antibodies.

4. You must learn how to _____ a logical argument.

5. We execute that _____ , we move to the next one.

Proverbs and Sayings

◇Always laugh when you can, it is cheap medicine.
  能笑的时候就笑，笑是便宜的药。

◇Think of exercise as medicine and take your daily prescription.
  把锻炼看作一种药物，每天服用你的处方。

◇To array a man's will against his sickness is the supreme art of medicine.
  用意志对抗疾病是医学的最高艺术。

题库

Appendix 1 Glossary

authority	/ɔːˈθɒrəti/	n.	权威；当局	7A
authorization	/ˌɔːθəraiˈzeiʃn/	n.	授权，认可；批准，委任	3A
authorize	/ˈɔːθəraiz/	vt.	批准；授权给；委托代替	3A
autonomous	/ɔːˈtɒnəməs/	adj.	自治的；自主的	9B
available	/əˈveiləbl/	adj.	可获得的；有空的	8B
awareness	/əˈweənəs/	n.	意识	7A

B

bacterial	/bækˈtiəriəl/	adj.	细菌的	7A
ban	/bæn/	n.	禁令	7A
barcode	/ˈbɑːkəud/	n.	条形码	10B
bark	/bɑːk/	n.	树皮	2A
barrier	/ˈbæriə (r) /	n.	障碍物，屏障；界线	6A
beneficial	/beniˈfiʃl/	adj.	有益的	4A
bid	/bid/	n.	出价	10B
biological	/ˌbaiəˈlɒdʒikl/	adj.	生物的；生物学的	3A
biopharma	/ˈbaiəufɑːmə/	n.	生物制药	6B
blanket	/ˈblæŋkit/	adj.	没有限制的	7A
blister	/ˈblistər/	n.	水疱	7B
boom	/buːm/	v.	迅速发展；激增；轰鸣	8A
		n.	激增；繁荣	8A
botany	/ˈbɒtəni/	n.	植物学	2A
branching	/ˈbræntʃiŋ/	n.	分支；分歧	3B
breakthrough	/ˈbreikθruː/	n.	突破	9A
breast-feeding	/brestˈfiːdiŋ/	vt.	用母乳喂养	7B
broad	/brɔːd/	adj.	宽的，辽阔的	9A

C

caplet	/ˈkæplət/	n.	囊片	7B
cardiology	/ˌkɑːdiˈɒlədʒi/	n.	心脏病学	8B
cardiovascular	/ˌkɑːdiəuˈvæskjələ (r) /	adj.	心血管的	4A
catalog	/ˈkætəlɒg/	n.	目录	9B
category	/ˈkætəgəri/	n.	范畴；类别，种类	3A
certified	/ˈsɜːtifaid/	adj.	被证实的；有保证的	8B
chain	/tʃein/	n.	链条；连锁商店；一系列	8A
channel	/ˈtʃænl/	n.	频道；途径；渠道	8B
chemotherapy	/ˌkiːməuˈθerəpi/	n.	[临床]化学疗法	1B
chiropractic	/kaiərəuˈpræktik/	n.	脊椎按摩疗法	1A
chloroquine	/ˈklɔːrə (ʊ) kwiːn/	n.	[药]氯喹	5B
chronic	/ˈkrɒnik/	adj.	慢性的	1B
civilization	/ˌsivəlaiˈzeiʃn/	n.	文明；文化	2A
classification	/ˌklæsifiˈkeiʃn/	n.	分类；类别，等级	3B
code	/kəud/	n.	密码；代码；行为准则	8B
commercialization	/kəˌmɜːʃəlaiˈzeiʃn/	n.	商品化，商业化	6A

续表

commitment	/kə'mitmənt/	n.	承诺；保证	10A
companion	/kəm'pæniən/	n.	伴侣；同伴；陪伴	8B
competent	/'kɒmpitənt/	adj.	胜任的；有能力的	9A
competitor	/kəm'petitə(r)/	n.	竞争者，对手；参赛者	8A
complementary	/ˌkɒmpli'mentri/	adj.	补足的；互补的	1A
component	/kəm'pəʊnənt/	nt.	组成部分	4A
compound	/'kɒmpaʊnd/	v.	合成；混合	2A
comprehensive	/ˌkɒmpri'hensiv/	adj.	综合的；广泛的	6A
compromise	/'kɒmprəmaiz/	vt.	妥协，让步；违背	8B
conceivably	/kən'si:vəbli/	adv.	可以想象的是	2A
condition	/kən'diʃən/	n.	情况	7A
conduct	/kən'dʌkt/	v.	进行，组织，实施	6B
confidential	/ˌkɒnfi'denʃl/	adj.	机密的	10B
conquer	/'kɒŋkə(r)/	vt.	战胜，征服；攻克	5B
consensus	/kən'sensəs/	n.	一致；舆论	4B
constraint	/kən'streint/	n.	限制；约束	8A
contaminate	/kən'tæmineit/	n.	污染	7A
contention	/kən'tenʃn/	n.	争论	4B
continuum	/kən'tinjuəm/	n.	连续体	10A
contract	/'kɒntrækt/	v.	收缩	1A
conventional	/kən'venʃənl/	adj.	符合习俗的，传统的	1B
cooperate	/kəʊ'ɒpəreit/	vi.	合作，配合；协力	9B
correlative	/kə'relətiv/	adj.	相关的	4A
cosmetic	/kɒz'metik/	n.	化妆品	9B
counsel	/'kaʊnsl/	vt.	建议；劝告	2B
		n.	法律顾问；忠告	2B
counterpart	/'kaʊntəpɑːt/	n.	配对物；极相似的人或物	2A
cramp	/kræmp/	n.	痉挛；绞痛	7B
cramped	/kræmpt/	adj.	狭窄的	7A
criteria	/krai'tiəriə/	n.	标准，条件	5A
crucial	/kruː'ʃl/	adj.	重要的；决定性的	10A
crude	/kruːd/	adj.	天然的，未加工的	4A
crystalline	/'kristəlain/	adj.	透明的；水晶般的	5B
cupping	/'kʌpiŋ/	n.	拔火罐	1A
curb	/kɜːb/	vt.	控制；抑制	7A
D				
default	/di'fɔːlt/	n.	默认；常规做法	6B
deliver	/di'livə(r)/	vt.	提供；交付；递送	6B
demonstrate	/'demənstreit/	vt.	证明；展示；论证	6A
dermatology	/ˌdɜːmə'tɒlədʒi/	n.	皮肤病学	8B
deterioration	/diˌtiəriə'reiʃn/	n.	恶化	10A
device	/di'vais/	n.	装置；设备	9B

续表

diabetes	/ˌdaɪə'biːtiːz/	n.	糖尿病；多尿症	2B
diagnosis	/ˌdaɪəg'nəʊsɪs/	n.	诊断	3A
diagnostics	/ˌdaɪəg'nɒstɪks/	n.	诊断学（用作单数）	1B
dictate	/dɪk'teɪt/	vt.	命令；口述	2A
dietary	/'daɪətəri/	adj.	饮食的；有关饮食的	8A
differ	/'dɪfə(r)/	vt.	使…相异；使…不同	9A
differentiate	/ˌdɪfə'renʃieɪt/	vt.	区分；区别；区别对待	8B
discipline	/'dɪsəplɪn/	n.	学科	4A
dispense	/dɪ'spens/	vt.	分配，分发	2B
dispenser	/dɪ'spensə(r)/	n.	药剂师；施与者	9A
disposal	/dɪ'spəʊzl/	n.	处理；支配	9B
disrupt	/dɪs'rʌpt/	vt.	破坏	1A
disruption	/dɪs'rʌpʃn/	n.	打乱，扰乱	10A
distribute	/dɪ'strɪbjuːt/	vt.	分配；把…分类	9A
distribution	/ˌdɪstrɪ'bjuːʃn/	n.	经销，分销；分发，分配	8A
diverse	/daɪ'vɜːs/	adj.	多种多样的	7A
domestically	/də'mestɪkli/	adv.	国内地	6B
dosage	/'dəʊsɪdʒ/	n.	剂量，用量	2B
dosing	/'dəʊsɪŋ/	n.	定量给料，配量	5A
draft	/drɑːft/	vt.	起草；制定	9B
drug	/drʌg/	n.	药；毒品	9A
E				
echelon	/'eʃəlɒn/	n.	等级；阶层	2A
e-commerce	/iː'kɒmɜːs/	n.	电子商务（同 e-business）	8A
efficacy	/'efɪkəsi/	n.	功效，效力	1B
elaborate	/i'læbəreɪt/	vt.	详细阐述；精心制作	8B
element	/'elɪmənt/	n.	元素；要素；原理	9A
elementary	/ˌeli'mentri/	adj.	基本的；初级的	2A
elusive	/i'luːsɪv/	adj.	难懂的	4B
embrace	/ɪm'breɪs/	vt.	拥抱；围绕	10A
emerging	/i'mɜːrdʒɪŋ/	adj.	新兴的；走向成熟的	1B
encompass	/ɪn'kʌmpəs/	vt.	包含；包围	1B
entity	/'entəti/	n.	实体	6B
eradicate	/i'rædikeɪt/	vt.	根除，根绝；消灭	5B
essential	/i'senʃl/	adj.	基本的；必要的；本质的	4A
ethnic	/'eθnɪk/	adj.	种族的；人种的	9B
evaluation	/iˌvæljuˈeɪʃn/	n.	评价；评估	6A
eventually	/i'ventʃuəli/	adv.	最后，终于	2A
evidence	/'evɪdəns/	n.	证据，证明	6A
		vt.	证明	6A
evolution	/ˌiːvə'luːʃn/	n.	进化；演变；发展	8A
evolve	/i'vɒlv/	vi.	发展；进化	1A

续表

exert	/ig'zɜːt/	v.	运用，发挥；施以影响	4A
expertise	/ˌekspɜː'tiːz/	n.	专门知识；专门技术	2B
expiration	/ˌekspə'reiʃn/	n.	呼气；终结；届期	3A
expound	/ik'spaʊnd/	v.	阐述；讲解	4A
extract	/'ekstrækt/	vt.	提取，提炼	4A
extraction	/ik'strækʃn/	n.	取出；抽出；抽出物	5B
F				
fabrication	/ˌfæbri'keiʃn/	n.	制造，建造	2A
facility	/fə'siləti/	n.	机构	7A
factor	/'fæktə(r)] /	n.	因素；要素；因子	8B
FDA	/ˌefdiː'ei/		美国食品和药物管理局	5A
fertile	/'fɜːtail/	adj.	能生育的	7A
flexibility	/ˌfleksə'biləti/	n.	灵活性；弹性；适应性	6B
flourish	/'flʌriʃ/	v.	繁荣；茂盛	9A
formula	/'fɔːmjələ/	n.	配方；准则	2A
formulate	/'fɔːmjuleit/	vt.	规划	9B
foundation	/faʊn'deiʃn/	n.	基础；地基	9A
framework	/'freimwɜːk/	n.	构架，框架；机制	8B
frightful	/'fraitfl/	adj.	可怕的；惊人的；非常的	3B
frontier	/'frʌntiə(r)/	n.	前沿	4B
G				
galenical	/gə'lenik(ə)l/	n.	天然制剂；盖仑制剂	2A
generate	/'dʒenəreit/	vt.	生殖；产生物理反应	3B
generation	/ˌdʒenə'reiʃn/	n.	一代；同辈；一代人	8A
generic	/dʒə'nerik/	adj.	类的；一般的；非商标的	3A
giant	/'dʒaiənt/	n.	巨人；巨兽；大公司	8A
		adj.	巨大的；伟大的	8A
governance	/'gʌvənəns/	n.	统治；管理；治理	8B
grocery	/'grəʊsəri/	n.	食品杂货店；食品杂货	3A
guild	/gild/	n.	协会，行会	2A
H				
haematology	/ˌhiːmə'tɒlədʒi/	n.	血液学	8B
hallmark	/'hɔːlmɑːk/	n.	特点；品质证明	1A
harmony	/'hɑːməni/	n.	和谐；协调	1A
harness	/'hɑːnis/	vt.	利用	10A
herbal	/'ɜːdl, 'hɜːdl/	adj.	草药的；草本的	1A
holistic	/həʊ'listik/	adj.	整体的	1A
hotspot	/'hɒtspɒt/	n.	热点	4A
hypertension	/ˌhaipə'tenʃn/	n.	高血压；过度紧张	3B
I				
identification	/ai,dentifi'keiʃn/	n.	鉴定，识别	4B
illegal	/i'liːgl/	adj.	非法的；违法的	9B

续表

immunization	/ˌimjunaiˈzeiʃn/	n.	免疫	2B
implement	/ˈimpliment/	vt.	使生效；贯彻；执行；实施	8A
implementation	/ˌimplimenˈteiʃn/	n.	实现；履行	9A
incentive	/inˈsentiv/	n.	动机；刺激	10A
incorporate	/inˈkɔːpəreit/	vt.	包含；把……合并	10A
indication	/ˌindiˈkeiʃn/	n.	适应证	4A
infection	/inˈfekʃən/	n.	感染，传染	7A
infrastructure	/ˈinfrəstrʌktʃə(r)/	n.	基础设施	10A
infusion	/inˈfjuːʒn/	n.	输液；灌输	1B
ingredient	/inˈgriːdiənt/	n.	原料；要素；组成部分	7B
inhibition	/ˌinhiˈbiʃn/	n.	抑制；压抑	5B
initiative	/iˈniʃətiv/	n.	（重要的）法案；倡议	7A
innovation	/ˌinəˈveiʃn/	n.	创新，革新	6A
innovative	/ˈinəveitiv/	adj.	革新的，创新的	1B
inspection	/inˈspekʃn/	n.	视察，检查	5A
instinct	/ˈinstiŋkt/	n.	本能，直觉；天性	2A
insurance	/inˈʃʊrəns/	n.	保险；保险费	2B
integration	/ˌintiˈgreiʃn/	n.	整合，集成	10B
intended	/inˈtendid/	adj.	有意的；打算中的	3A
intensity	/inˈtensəti/	n.	强烈；剧烈；强度	8A
interact	/ˌintərˈækt/	vt. /vi.	互相影响；互相作用	3A
interaction	/ˌintərˈækʃn/	n.	相互作用，相互影响	9A
intern	/ˈintɜːn/	n.	实习生，实习医师	2B
intervention	/ˌintəˈvenʃn/	n.	介入；调停	1A
inventory	/ˈinvəntri/	n.	存货，存货清单	2B
investigational	/inˌvestiˈgeiʃnəl/	adj.	试验性的	6A
L				
lag	/læg/	n.	落后；迟延	6B
legend	/ˈledʒənd/	n.	传奇；传说；说明	2A
lethal	/ˈliːθl/	adj.	致命的，致死的	3B
leverage	/ˈliːvəridʒ/	v.	利用	4B
license	/ˈlaisns/	n.	许可证，执照	6B
likelihood	/ˈlaiklihʊd/	n.	可能性，可能	6A
liver	/ˈlivər/	n.	肝脏	7B
looming	/ˈluːmiŋ/	adj.	（不希望的事情）逼近的	7A
M				
macromolecule	/ˈmækrə(ʊ)ˈmɒlikjuːl/	n.	高分子；［化学］大分子	3B
majority	/məˈdʒɒrəti/	n.	多数	6B
management	/ˈmænidʒmənt/	n.	管理	10A
mandate	/ˈmændeit/	vt.	授权；托管	5A
manual	/ˈmænjuəl/	adj.	手控的；用手的	10B
manufacture	/ˌmænjuˈfæktʃə(r)/	n.	制造；产品；制造业	6A

续表

manufacture	/ˌmænjuˈfæktʃə(r)/	vt.	制造；加工	6A
margin	/ˈmɑːdʒin/	n.	边缘；利润；页边的空白	3A
market	/ˈmɑːkit/	vt.	在市场上出售	9A
mass	/mæs/	n.	块；民众；大量；质量	3B
		adj.	群众的；集中的	3B
massage	/məˈsɑːʒ/	n.	按摩，推拿	1A
medical	/ˈmedikl/	adj.	医学的；药的；内科的	4A
medication	/ˌmediˈkeiʃn/	n.	药物；药物治疗	1B
medications	/ˌmediˈkeiʃn/	n.	药物；药物治疗（处理）	3A
medicinal	/məˈdisinl/	adj.	药的；药用的；治疗的	4A
meridian	/məˈridiən/	n.	中医经脉；经线	1A
microcosm	/ˈmaikrəukɒzəm/	n.	微观世界；缩图	1A
migrate	/maiˈgreit/	vt.	迁徙；移动	7A
milestone	/ˈmailstəun/	n.	里程碑，划时代的事件	6A
minor	/ˈmainər/	adj.	次要的；轻微的	7B
misleading	/ˌmisˈliːdiŋ/	adj.	误导的；让人产生错误观念的	6A
mission	/ˈmiʃn/	n.	使命，任务	9A
misuse	/ˌmisˈjuːz/	n.	误用；滥用	7A
modification	/ˌmɒdifiˈkeiʃn/	n.	修改，修正	1B
molecular	/məˈlekjələ(r)/	adj.	分子的；由分子组成的	3B
molecule	/ˈmɒlikjuːl/	n.	[化学]分子；微粒	3B
monitor	/ˈmɒnitə(r)/	vt.	监控	9B
motive	/ˈməutiv/	n.	动机，目的	9A
municipality	/mjuːˌnisiˈpæləti/	n.	市政当局；自治市或区	9B
N				
nationwide	/ˌneiʃnˈwaid/	adj.	全国范围的；全国性的	8A
		adv.	在全国范围内	8A
nature	/ˈneitʃə(r)/	n.	性质；本性	4A
navigate	/ˈnævigeit/	vt.	进行；行驶；航行	6A
necessity	/nəˈsesəti/	n.	必然；必要；必需品	8A
negative	/ˈnegətiv/	n.	负的；阴性的	1A
non-prescription	/ˌnɑːnpriˈskripʃn/	adj.	非处方的	3A
normality	/nɔːˈmæləti/	n.	常态；正常的形势	8A
O				
objective	/əbˈdʒektiv/	n.	目标；目的	8B
oncology	/ɒŋˈkɒlədʒi/	n.	肿瘤学	8B
onerous	/ˈəunərəs/	adj.	繁重的，麻烦的	6A
opt	/ɒpt/	vi.	选择	1B
optimal	/ˈɒptiməl/	adj.	最佳的；最理想的	1A
optional	/ˈɒpʃənl/	adj.	可选择的，随意的	4B
optometrist	/ɒpˈtɒmətrist/	n.	验光师；视力测定者	3A
originate	/əˈridʒineit/	vi.	发源	1A

续表

outpatient	/ˈaʊtpeiʃnt/	n.	门诊病人	7A
overarching	/ˌəʊvərˈɑːtʃiŋ/	adj.	总体的；首要的	10A
overburdened	/ˌəʊvəˈbɜːdənd/	adj.	负担过重的	10A
overdose	/ˈəʊvədəʊs/	n.	药量过多	7B
overdue	/ˌəʊvəˈdʒuː/	adj.	早该发生的	7A
oversee	/ˌəʊvəˈsiː/	vt.	监督；审查	2B
overt	/əʊˈvɜːt/	adj.	明显的	1A
over-the-counter	/ˌəʊvəðə ˈkaʊntə(r)/	adj.	非处方的	2B
overuse	/ˌəʊvəˈjuːs/	n.	过度使用	7A
P				
pain	/pein/	n.	疼痛	7B
pandemic	/pænˈdemik/	n.	流行病	4B
parallel	/ˈpærəlel/	vt.	使…与…平行	2A
parasite	/ˈpærəsait/	n.	寄生虫；食客	5B
participate	/pɑːˈtisipeit/	vi.	参与，参加；分享	9B
patent	/ˈpæt(ə)nt/	n.	专利	4B
pathway	/ˈpɑːθwei/	n.	道；路径；神经通路	3B
peculiar	/piˈkjuːliə(r)/	adj.	奇怪的；不寻常的	8B
permeate	/ˈpɜːmieit/	vt.	渗透，透过；弥漫	1A
perspective	/pəˈspektiv/	n.	观点；角度	6A
pest	/pest/	n.	害虫；讨厌的人	8B
pharma	/ˈfɑːmə/	n.	制药公司	5A
pharmaceutical	/ˌfɑːməˈsuːtikl/	adj.	制药（学）的	2A
		n.	药物	2A
pharmacist	/ˈfɑːməsist/	n.	药剂师	2A
pharmacological	/ˌfɑːməkəˈlɒdʒikl/	adj.	药理学的	3B
pharmacology	/ˌfɑːməˈkɒlədʒi/	n.	药物学，药理学	2B
pharmacopoeia	/ˌfɑːməkəˈpiːə/	n.	药典	9A
pharmacy	/ˈfɑːməsi/	n.	药房；配药学，药剂学	2A
phenomenon	/fəˈnɒminən/	n.	现象（复数 phenomena）	1A
philosopher	/fəˈlɒsəfə(r)/	n.	哲学家	2A
philosophy	/fəˈlɒsəfi/	n.	哲学；哲理；人生观	1A
physician	/fiˈziʃn/	n.	医师，内科医师	2A
physiology	/ˌfiziˈɒlədʒi/	n.	生理学；生理机能	5B
platform	/ˈplætfɔːm/	n.	平台；讲台；站台	8A
portfolio	/pɔːtˈfəʊliəʊ/	n.	组合；投资组合	8B
positive	/ˈpɒzətiv/	adj.	正的，阳性的	1A
practitioner	/prækˈtiʃənə(r)/	n.	开业者，从业者，执业医生	3A
precise	/priˈsais/	adj.	精确的；明确的	10A
preclinical	/priːˈklinik(ə)l/	adj.	临床前的	5A
pregnant	/ˈpregnənt/	adj.	怀孕的	7B
premature	/ˈpremətʃər/	n.	早产儿	7A

医药大学堂
WWW.YIYAODXT.COM

续表

premenstrual	/ˌpriːˈmenstruəl/	adj.	月经前的；经期前的	7B
premise	/ˈpremis/	n.	前提，假定	1A
prescribe	/priˈskraib/	vt.	开处方	7A
prescription	/priˈskripʃn/	n.	药方；指示	2A
presence	/ˈprezns/	n.	出席；在场；存在	8B
prevailing	/priˈveiliŋ/	adj.	流行的；盛行很广的	5B
pricing	/ˈpraisiŋ/	n.	定价；计价	8B
		vt.	给……定价；标价	8B
priest	/priːst/	n.	牧师；神父	2A
principal	/ˈprinsəpl/	adj.	主要的	5B
priority	/praiˈɒrəti/	n.	优先；优先权	6A
processing	/ˈprəʊsesiŋ/	n.	加工	4A
procurement	/prəˈkjuəmənt/	n.	采购，购买	8B
professional	/prəˈfeʃnl/	adj.	专业的；职业的	9A
property	/ˈprɒpəti/	n.	性质，性能	1A
propose	/prəˈpəʊz/	vt.	提出，计划	6A
proposition	/ˌprɒpəˈziʃn/	n.	提议；建议；任务	8A
prospect	/ˈprɒspekt/	n.	可能性；希望；前景	8A
protocol	/ˈprəʊtəkɒl/	n.	协议；方案	1A
psychiatrist	/saiˈkaiətrist/	n.	精神病学家，精神病医生	3A
purification	/ˌpjuərifiˈkeiʃn/	n.	提纯	4B
R				
radiation	/ˌreidiˈeiʃn/	n.	辐射；放射物	1B
rash	/ræʃ/	n.	（皮肤）皮疹	7B
reaction	/riˈækʃn/	n.	反应，感应	9B
readmission	/ˌriːədˈmiʃn/	n.	再入院	10A
rear	/riə(r)/	vt.	喂养；培养	7A
reassure	/ˌriːəˈʃʊə(r)/	vt.	使……安心；打消……的疑虑	8A
recognize	/ˈrekəgnaiz/	v.	认出；承认	10A
recommendation	/ˌrekəmenˈdeiʃn/	n.	推荐；介绍；正式建议	8A
recruit	/riˈkruːt/	v.	征募；聘用	6B
redden	/ˈredn/	v.	（使）变红	7B
referral	/riˈfɜːrəl/	n.	转诊	10A
reflection	/riˈflekʃn/	n.	反映	4A
reflexology	/ˌriːfleksˈɒlədʒi/	n.	［心理］反射学；（按摩脚部的）反射疗法	1A
regarding	/riˈgɑːdiŋ/	prep.	关于；就……而论	3A
registration	/ˌredʒiˈstreiʃn/	n.	注册；登记；挂号	6B
regulation	/ˌregjuˈleiʃn/	n.	章程；规则；规章制度	8A
reimbursement	/ˌriːimˈbɜːsmənt/	n.	报销；偿还	10A
relevant	/ˈreləvənt/	adj.	相关的；切题的	9B
remedy	/ˈremədi/	n.	疗法	1A

医药大学堂
WWW.YIYAODXT.COM

续表

remote	/rɪˈməʊt/	adj.	遥远的；远程的	10A
restriction	/rɪˈstrɪkʃn/	n.	制约因素；限制规定	8A
retail	/ˈriːteɪl/	n.	零售	8A
		vt.	零售；零卖；转述	8A
revaluation	/ˌriːˌvæljuˈeɪʃn/	n.	重新估价；再评价	4A
revenue	/ˈrevənjuː/	n.	税收收入；财政收入	5A
revere	/rɪˈvɪə(r)/	vt.	敬畏；尊敬；崇敬	2A
rigorous	/ˈrɪɡərəs/	adj.	严格的，严厉的；严酷的	6A
robotics	/rəʊˈbɒtɪks/	n.	机器人技术	10B
rodent	/ˈrəʊdnt/	n.	啮齿目动物	5B
roughly	/ˈrʌfli/	adv.	大致；大约；粗糙地	8A
route	/ruːt/	n.	途径，渠道；路线	6B
routine	/ruːˈtiːn/	adj.	常规的，例行的	10B
S				
scanner	/ˈskænə/	n.	扫描仪	10B
scope	/skəʊp/	n.	范围	10A
scraping	/ˈskreɪpɪŋ/	n.	刮痧	1A
screening	/ˈskriːnɪŋ/	n.	筛查，筛检	2B
scribe	/skraɪb/	vt.	写下，记下	2A
scripture	/ˈskrɪptʃə(r)/	n.	经文；（大写）圣经	1A
sector	/ˈsektə/	n.	部门	10B
self-treatment	/selfˈtriːtmənt/	n.	自我治疗	7A
simultaneous	/ˌsɪmlˈteɪniəs/	adj.	同时的；同时发生的	6B
skeletal	/ˈskelətl/	adj.	骨骼的；骨瘦如柴的	3B
skeptical	/ˈskeptɪkl/	adj.	怀疑的	4B
smoothen	/ˈsmuːðən/	vt.	使平滑；使平和	8B
soothing	/ˈsuːðɪŋ/	adj.	抚慰的；使人宽心的	2A
spoiled	/spɔɪld/	adj.	（尤指小孩）被宠坏的	3B
sponsor	/ˈspɒnsə(r)/	n.	赞助商；主办者	6A
		vt.	赞助；发起	6A
stakeholder	/ˈsteɪkhəʊldə(r)/	n.	利益相关者	7A
state-level	/steɪtˈlevl/	adj.	国家级	7A
statistical	/stəˈtɪstɪkl/	adj.	统计的；统计学的	6B
streamline	/ˈstriːmlaɪn/	vt.	组织；集成	10B
stretch	/stretʃ/	v.	延长；伸展；延续	6A
stretched	/stretʃt/	adj.	拉伸的；延伸的	10A
stringent	/ˈstrɪndʒənt/	adj.	严格的；严厉的	6A
stroke	/strəʊk/	n.	中风	10A
stuff	/stʌf/	n.	东西；材料；填充物	9A
submit	/səbˈmɪt/	vt.	呈递；提交	5A
substance	/ˈsʌbstəns/	n.	物质；实质；资产；主旨	3A
suite	/swiːt/	n.	（一套）套间	10A

续表

sulphonamides	/ˌsʌlfə'næmaid/	n.	磺胺；磺胺类药剂	3B
superbug	/'suːpəbʌg/	n.	超级细菌	7A
supervise	/'suːpərvaiz/	v.	监督；管理；指导	2B
surpass	/sə'pɑːs/	vt.	超越	10B
survival	/sə'vaivl/	n.	（在困境中的）生存	4A
swamp	/swɒmp/	n.	沼泽	2A
swelling	/'sweliŋ/	n.	肿胀	7B
symptom	/'simptəm/	n.	［临床］症状；征兆	1A
synthetic	/sin'θetik/	adj.	综合的；合成的，人造的	3B
		n.	合成物	3B
systematical	/ˌsistə'mætikl/	adj.	系统的	4A
		T		
tackle	/'tækl/	vt.	处理（难题或局面）	7A
tailor	/'teilə(r)/	n.	裁缝	3A
		v.	专门制作；调整；迎合	3A
target	/'tɑːgit/	v.	把…作为目标；面向	3B
		n.	（攻击的）对象；靶子	3B
territory	/'terətri/	n.	领土	4A
theoretical	/ˌθiə'retikl/	adj.	理论的；理论上的	4A
therapeutic	/ˌθerə'pjuːtik/	adj.	治疗的	1A
therapeutically	/ˌθerə'pjuːtikli/	adv.	在治疗上；有疗效地	3B
tier	/tiə(r)/	n.	等级；层	10A
toxic	/'tɒksik/	adj.	有毒的；中毒的	3B
toxicity	/tɒk'sisəti/	n.	毒性	5A
toxicology	/ˌtɒksi'kɒlədʒi/	n.	毒物学，毒理学	4B
traction	/'trækʃn/	n.	牵引	4B
transform	/'trænsfɔːm/	vt.	改变；转换	10B
transition	/træn'ziʃn/	n.	过渡；转变	5A
transparent	/'trænspærənt/	adj.	透明的；清澈的	8A
trial	/'traiəl/	n.	试验；审讯	1B
trials	/'traiəl/	n.	试验；审讯；努力；磨炼	3B
		U		
undergo	/ˌʌndə'gəʊ/	vt.	经历，经受	5A
underlying	/ˌʌndə'laiiŋ/	adj.	潜在的；根本的	1A
		V		
vehicle	/'viːəkl/	n.	媒介；工具；车辆	6A
veterinarian	/ˌvetəri'neəriən/	n.	兽医	3A
vial	/'vaiəl/	n.	小瓶；药水瓶	10B
virtual	/'vɜːtʃuəl/	adj.	虚拟的	10A
vital	/'vaitl/	adj.	至关重要的；生死攸关的	3A
		W		
weapon	/'wepən/	n.	手段	4A

续表

wearable	/ˈweərəbl/	n.	可穿戴设备	10A
wellness	/ˈwelnəs/	n.	健康	3A
wholesaler	/ˈhəʊlseilə(r)/	n.	批发商	3A
widespread	/ˈwaidspred/	adj.	普遍的；广泛的	7A
worship	/ˈwɜːʃip/	vt.	崇拜；尊敬	2A

Appendix 2 Keys & Translation for Reference

Unit 1

Keys to Exercises

Warming-up

1. D; 2. B; 3. A; 4. C

Reading A

Task 1

1. Yin and Yang, Qi and The Five Elements are the basic philosophies of Traditional Chinese Medicine.

2. Harmony between yin and yang is thought to promote health. But imbalance is thought to result in disease.

3. The concept was first noted in the oldest TCM scriptures, named the 'Internal Scripture'.

4. All things in the universe can be classified under different properties, functions or appearances represented by metal, wood, water, fire or earth.

5. Traditional Chinese Medicine principles can help you strengthen your holistic health and wellness. It can guide you as you develop a healthier lifestyle that connects the pillars of physical, emotional, environmental, nutritional, and spiritual health.

Task 2

1. g; 2. j; 3. i; 4. b; 5. h; 6. a; 7. c; 8. f; 9. d; 10. e

Task 3

1. complement; 2. originated; 3. intervene; 4. symptoms; 5. positive

Task 4

1. Traditional Chinese Medicine dates back more than 2,500 years and has evolved and been perfected ever since.

2. The Chinese believed that Qi permeated everything and linked their bodies' to the surrounding environment.

3. Harmony between yin and yang is thought to promote health.

4. The Five Elements consist of metal, wood, water, fire and earth.

5. Traditional Chinese Medicine principles can help you strengthen your holistic health and wellness.

Listening & Speaking

Task 1

Diseases

Michael: Lisa, what happened, dear? Why are you sad?

Lisa: Michael, my best friend Rachel didn't come to school today. She is sick. She is suffering from chickenpox.

Michael：Oh that's so sad.

Lisa：Michael, how did Rachel get chickenpox. Can you explain me that?

Michael：Sure, but first you should know that diseases can be of two types: communicable and non-communicable. There are some diseases that cannot be spread from one person to another. They are called non-communicable diseases like the heart diseases, blood pressure.

Lisa：And what about the communicable disease? How are they caused?

Michael：Communicable diseases can spread from an infected person to a healthy person.

Lisa：But what causes these diseases?

Michael：Communicable diseases are caused by agents like the bacteria, fungi, protozoa and the virus. Viruses cause diseases like AIDS, chickenpox and common cold.

Lisa：How do these agents spread?

Michael：They spread by air, food, carriers, water and direct contact. The tuberculosis, chickenpox and common cold can be spread through air.

Lisa：How can we prevent these diseases?

Michael：We should eat clean food. Another way is to get vaccinated in the form of injection or oral drops. We have vaccines against many infectious diseases including chickenpox.

Lisa：Ok, I see. Thank you Michael!

1. F; 2. F; 3. T; 4. T; 5. F

Task 2

Western and Eastern Medicine

Lisa：Hi Hardy! Can you tell me what the L. Ac after your name stands for?

Hardy：Of cause. I'm a licensed acupuncturist, that's what the L. Ac stands for. So, what's the matter with you?

Lisa：I'm not sleeping well, and I've been super tired for a long time.

Hardy：Have you seen a doctor before?

Lisa：Yes. I have gone to a general practice physician, and she prescribed me a common anti-anxiety medicine I have never taken. I'm not sure if I will experience side-effects.

Hardy：OK. Is there anything that upsets you recently?

Lisa：Yes. I lost my job, but lack the competitive skills to find a new one.

Hardy：Your job loss is a root cause of your issues. I'll book you for regular acupuncture treatments to treat insomnia and stress. You should gain your mental health back first.

Lisa：Sounds good. I find there is difference between Western and Eastern Medicine. It seems that you take a holistic approach to medicine, while my previous physician took a reductionist approach.

Hardy：Yes. Western medicine views the human body as a machine, while alternative or eastern medicine evaluates the entire person, physical (body) and non-physical (mind), and seeks to heal any imbalances between the two.

1. B; 2. D; 3. C; 4. A; 5. D

Task 3

The combination of Traditional Chinese Medicine (TCM) and Western Medicine has been a highlight of China's prevention and control of the novel coronavirus disease (COVID-19). It was a significant guarantee for the current success the country has achieved in the epidemic control, as well as a Chinese strategy to share with the international community.

1. combination；2. prevention；3. control；4. achieved；5. strategy

Reading B

Task 1

1. D；2. B；3. A；4. C；5. D

Task 2

1. 西医以临床研究和方法为基础，包括使用外科手术作为治疗方法。

2. 在这个国家，大多数患有慢性疾病的人都是西医给与诊断。

3. 循证治疗计划可能包括处方药物、手术、输液和其他常规程序和疗法。

4. 临床试验是一种用于确定治疗干预措施效果和结果的对照研究，治疗干预措施包括药物、新的医疗程序，甚至生活方式的改变。

5. 因此，如果根据你的调查，你认为你应该接受一些特定的检查，要向你的医生询问这些检查，这很重要。而不是假设这些检查已经进行过或者就认为它们是合适的。

Practical Writing

Job Posting

Pharmacist

Tired of working in a hospital? Come work at Sun Health Medical where you can make a difference!

The Company：

Sun Health Medical, located in Fuzhou Industrial Park, was set up in 2007. We have been offering International medical services for both the local and expatriate communities in Fuzhou.

The Position：

We are presently seeking an enthusiastic, experienced, self-motivated licensed pharmacist with a background in hospital pharmacy to join our dynamic team. You will also be outgoing and team oriented.

Salary is 4000-6000 RMB monthly.

Requirements：

· College diploma or above with tertiary qualifications in pharmacy

· Proficiency with Microsoft Word and Excel.

Those with experience in hospital pharmacy are preferred, and those who are proficient in spoken English will be better paid.

WHY SHOULD YOU APPLY?

· Top benefits.

· Excellent growth and advancement opportunities.

If you have the skillset described above, and are ready to take on a new and exciting challenge, then please email your application to：

sunhealthmedical@ email. com

Grammar Tips

Task 1

1. 名词, 副词; 2. 动词, 名词; 3. 代词, 介词; 4. 连词, 动词; 5. 代词, 数词; 6. 感叹词, 动词; 7. 冠词, 副词; 8. 代词, 介词; 9. 冠词, 连词; 10. 代词, 形容词

Task 2

1. C; 2. C; 3. D; 4. A; 5. D; 6. D; 7. C; 8. C; 9. A; 10. B

Supplementary Reading

1. T; 2. F; 3. F; 4. F; 5. T

VocabularyTips

1. diagnostic; 2. biology; 3. herbicide; 4. acme; 5. diaphragm

Translation for Reference

课文 A

中 医

中医通常也被称为"东方医学",起源于古代中国大陆。中医可追溯到 2500 多年前,并从那时起不断发展完善。但中医到底是什么呢?要理解中医,首先要从其基本理论开始。

阴阳

中医道法自然。中医的基本前提是,我们的身体是我们周围世界和宇宙的一个缩影。阴阳是东方科学和中医的基础。阴阳概念是指对立的力量实际上是互补,(互为)根本,需要在平衡、和谐中存在,以达到最佳的健康状态。举例:

· 光明与黑暗

· 积极与消极

· 火与水

· 善与恶

· 男与女

· 扩张与收缩

可以这样认为。没有光就不存在阴影。就像许多现代超级英雄电影一样——如果没有邪恶就没有善良。中医阴阳学说的基本前提是这些看似对立的力量需要平衡和和谐地存在。阴阳和谐就可以促进健康。但是阴阳不平衡就会导致疾病。

气

气(读为"Chee"),通常被定义为流经所有生物体的"生命力"。中国人认为,气渗透于万物,并使我们的身体与周围环境联系在一起。

气的概念在传统中医中根深蒂固。最古老的中医典籍《内经》中最早记载这一概念。认为气在我们的身体里通过经络进行循行。经络气滞、中断或不平衡就会产生疾病症状或明显的疾病。

气在我们体内正常循行身体就健康。因此，中医的主要目标是调气，使得气在我们体内正常循行。

五行

东方医学的另一个重要理论就是所谓的"五行"。五行由金、木、水、火、土组成。五种物质代表不同的功能、属性或性状，宇宙间万物并以此进行归类。五行概念用来描述所有自然现象之间的相互作用和关系，包括人类生命的各个阶段，并解释身体的功能及它在健康或疾病期间的变化。

医生制定各种方案来治疗潜在的健康状况的根源。这些方案包括对营养、饮食的干预，草药疗法和各种身心练习。这些疗法包括针灸、拔火罐、治疗性按摩、刮痧、反射疗法、骨复位、脊椎指压疗法、呼吸、锻炼和自卫训练。

古老的中医观念强调自然的、预防性的方法。传统中医理论的核心是，如果采取了正确的纠正和预防措施对身体是有帮助的。中医理论知识有助于提升整体健康，指导你养成一种更健康的生活方式，这种生活方式能把人们健康的主要因素如身体、情感、环境、营养和精神等连接起来。

课文 B

西 医

西医以临床研究和方法为基础，包括使用外科手术作为治疗方法。西医包括各种常见的医学治疗方法，如：手术、化疗、放射和物理治疗。在美国，大多数人从医生、护士、医师助理（PAs）及其他医疗服务提供者那里获得大部分医疗服务，提供医疗服务的场所有医院、诊所或医生办公室等。大多数人听到"医疗保健"这个词时，想到的就是这个系统。通常该系统被称为"西医"，也被称为"对抗疗法""常见疗法"或"传统疗法"。西医是美国和西方世界最常见的医疗保健形式。

西医擅长检测和诊断。在美国，大多数患有慢性疾病的人都是西医给予诊断。西医治疗长期病患者的目标是：

- 诊断疾病
- 阻止疾病进展
- 缓解与疾病相关的症状
- 防止疾病传播
- 治愈疾病（如果能够治愈）
- 提高生活质量

西医是循证医学

西医医生根据对照的科学研究来决定哪种治疗对他们的病人最有帮助。这种方法被称为循证医学。循证治疗计划可能包括处方药物、手术、输液和其他常规程序和疗法。由于了解生活方式和身体健康之间的联系，对许多有慢性健康问题的美国人来说西医医生也更普遍地鼓励改变生活方式——尤其是饮食和锻炼。

如何决定治疗是否是循证疗法？临床试验是一种用于确定治疗干预措施效果和结果的对照研究，治疗干预措施包括药物、新的医疗程序，甚至生活方式的改变。临床试验增加了与疾病预防、诊断和治疗相关的医学知识。临床试验为病人提供了使用新兴的创新疗法进行治疗的机会。

在某些情况下，病人从临床试验中获益良多。然而，临床试验总是会给参与者带来伤害的风险，而临床试验的结果，比如美国食品和药物管理局批准的新药，通常会对未来的病人有益。参加临床试验是一个需要认真考虑的决定，并与你的医生和其他值得信任的医疗保健和支持团队成员进行讨论。

西医：化验室和诊断学

西医使用如实验室检测和成像扫描的诊断手段，在监测和评估疾病状态和进展方面发挥着关键作用。这些试验极为重要，因为它们提供了有关疾病状态变化的客观生物数据。这些诊断测试的结果可以帮助您了解，在您的医疗保健计划中哪些是有效的（哪些是无效的），并有助于你和你的医疗服务提供者作出明智的决策。请记住，医生不能也不应该为了监控一种特定的疾病而要求病人去做每一种检查，不同的医生可能会选择要求不同的检查。因此，如果根据你的调查，你认为你应该接受一些特定的检查，要向你的医生询问这些检查是很重要的。而不是假定这些检查已经进行过或者就认为它们是合适的。要始终保持试验检测结果的记录。

补充阅读

人类疾病

根据医生或科学家所需要的信息，疾病有很多种分类方式。

流行病学和流行病

流行病学是一种根据其影响的人口群体或传播方式的疾病分类方法，是非常重要的一门科学。公共卫生官员利用流行病学进行研究和管理社会对疾病的反应。

流行病学家试图预测在一个人口受到一种常见情况（如未经处理的饮用水）影响的地区发生一种或多种疾病的可能性有多大。这些预测是建立在数学公式的基础上的，这些数学公式决定了在特定情况下某一结果的概率。

流行病学家还关注流行性疾病，即在相对较短的时间内感染许多人或整个人口的疾病。历史上发生过许多毁灭性的流行病，从中世纪欧洲的鼠疫，到1918—1919年的流感大流行（全球流行病），再到目前困扰世界大部分地区的新冠肺炎。当一种疾病年复一年地、顽固地存在于同一地区时，它就被称为地方病。例如，黄热病是热带南美洲和非洲的地方病。

急性病与慢性病

疾病通常被定义为急性或慢性。急性病发病快，大多数疗程相对较短，在此期间症状可能是轻微或严重。普通感冒是一种相对温和的急性病，病程相当短。严重急性呼吸系统综合征（SARS）也会迅速发作，但SARS可以迅速变得非常严重，甚至致命。慢性疾病发病缓慢，持续时间长，可持续数年。类风湿关节炎是一种病程很长的慢性疾病。有些疾病，如支气管炎，有急性和慢性两种形式。

传染性和非传染性疾病

疾病分类最重要的方法之一是区分传染性疾病和非传染性疾病。传染性疾病是由活的生物体引起的，如细菌、真菌、原生动物、病毒和寄生虫。无论病原体是什么，它都能在"宿主"体内存活——换句话说，它是有传染性的。如果它能传染给另一个人，它也是会传染的。非传染性疾病不是由生物引起的；因为它们不会从一个人传到另一个人，所以它们是非传染性的。

器官系统的疾病

通常，疾病是根据受影响的器官或器官系统进行分类。包括呼吸系统疾病（肺炎）、心血管系统疾病（冠状动脉疾病）、神经系统疾病（多发性硬化症）和内分泌系统疾病（糖尿病）等。

局部性疾病与全身性疾病

疾病及其相关体征和症状可根据其在体内的传播程度进一步加以区分。局部的疾病或症状局限于特定部位或单一器官系统，而全身性疾病则影响全身。这是治疗疾病中的一个重要因素。例如，如果感染的伤口限于伤口部位，可以用局部抗生素药膏治疗。如果感染侵入更深的组织并扩散到血液中，感染的有机体就会被带到身体的每一个器官。治疗这种情况，医生必须开口服或注射的全身治疗药物，这种治疗药物可以进入血液，并在所有受感染部位对抗感染。

Unit 2

Keys to Exercises

Warming-up

1. C; 2. A; 3. D; 4. B

Reading A

Task 1

1. Ancient man learned from instinct, from observation of birds and beasts and apply cool water, leaf, dirt, or mud to soothe people.

2. Ancient Babylonian methods find counterpart in today's modern pharmaceutical, medical, and spiritual care of the sick.

3. Because Shen Nong examined many herbs, barks, and roots brought in from the fields, swamps, and woods, and wrote the first Pen T-Sao, or native herbal, recording 365 drugs, he was is still worshiped by native Chinese drug guilds as their patron god.

4. Theophrastus (about 300 B. C.), among the greatest early Greek philosophers and natural scientists, is called the "father of botany".

5. "Galenicals" refers to the class of pharmaceuticals compounded by mechanical means.

Task 2

1. g; 2. h; 3. b; 4. j; 5. i; 6. e; 7. a; 8. c; 9. d; 10. f

Task 3

1. prescribe; 2. compounding; 3. pharmacist; 4. soothe; 5. counterpart

Task 4

1. Ancient man learned from instinct, from observation of birds and beasts.

2. Babylon provides the earliest known record of practice of the art of the apothecary.

3. Chinese Pharmacy, according to legend, stems from Shen Nong.

4. He described over 500 plant species and devised an advanced classification scheme for plants.

5. His principles of preparing and compounding medicines ruled in the Western world for 1,500 years.

Listening & Speaking

Task 1

What's Your Major?

Ajay: Thanks for meeting up today, guys. I'm happy that I've met so many other exchange students already.

Jana: Yeah, we're all in the same boat, so let's try to support one another throughout the semester.

Ajay: Are we taking any of the same classes?

Lee: I think we all have different majors, so we might not be in any of the same classes.

Akinyi: What's your major, Lee?

Lee: My major is nursing. How about you?

Akinyi: Mine is quite different. I'm majoring in TCM, that's Traditional Chinese Medicine. I like traditional Chinese culture.

Ajay: And my major is clinical medicine. How about you, Jana? What's your major?

Jana: I'm studying pharmacy. I want to be a pharmacist.

1. T; 2. F; 3. F; 4. F; 5. T

Task 2

Why do You Want to be a Pharmacist?

Lee: Why do you want to be a pharmacist, Jana?

Jana: Well, I really like the sciences but I also really like helping people, And I hope to combine those two.

Ajay: To be a doctor can combine these two.

Jana: Yes, that's right. While I was considering my major, one of my good friends Dustin said, "Jana, you want to help people and you're good at chemistry why don't you go into pharmacy?"

Akinyi: So you take his advice?

Jana: Yes, I think pharmacists are the last line between patients and medications that can be deadly if taken incorrectly.

Lee: Where does a pharmacist work? Also in the hospital?

Jana: Not exactly. He can work at the inpatient department at the hospital or he can do more of outpatient pharmacy services or he can work at community pharmacy, such as Walgreens or even in a company.

Ajay: I think pharmacist should also be competent to communicate effectively with a patient.

Jana: Yes, that's what I like to do.

Lee: In a word, we are all part of a health care team in the future.

1. C; 2. B; 3. D; 4. D; 5. A

Task 3

Whenever a doctor writes a prescription for a drug or treatment, a <u>pharmacist</u> is the person who <u>measures</u> out the medication and makes sure a patient knows how to take it safely. And while <u>filling</u> a prescription often means a visit to the local drug store or grocery store, pharmacists also work in <u>hospitals</u>.

Typically, pharmacists spend most of the day standing at a counter, preparing and dispensing medication. They may also personalize or "compound" the medication, though that is now less common than it used to be.

1. pharmacist; 2. measures; 3. filling; 4. hospitals; 5. compound

Reading B

Task 1

1. C; 2. A; 3. D; 4. C; 5. D

Task 2

1. 药剂师还可能进行健康检查，提供免疫接种，监督给病人的药物治疗，并就健康的生活方式提供建议。

2. 他们给病人分发药物，并回答病人关于处方、非处方药或病人可能存在的任何健康问题。

3. 他们建议给病人用药，并监督药物的剂量和时间。

4. 要做到这一点，他们必须能够评估病人的需求和医生的指令，并有广泛的知识，能了解药物效果以及在合适的情况给予特定药物。

5. 药剂师还必须在整个职业生涯中接受继续教育课程，以跟上药学的最新进展。

Practical Writing

Singapore Visa Application Form

Full name   Liu Yang   Chinese characters   刘洋

Date and place of birth   June 6, 1995, Shanghai

Gender   Male   Marital status   Single

Nationality   Chinese   Nationality at birth   Chinese

Permanent address   No. 50 Nanjing Road, Shanghai

Present address   No. 50 Nanjing Road, Shanghai

Occupation   Student

Reason for visit   Travel

Proposed duration of stay   5 days

Signature   刘洋   Date   August 17, 2019

Grammar Tips

Task 1

1. 主语，定语; 2. 谓语，状语; 3. 定语，表语; 4. 宾语，状语; 5. 谓语，主语; 6. 主语，表语; 7. 谓语，宾语; 8. 宾语，定语; 9. 插入语，状语; 10. 形式主语，表语，宾补

Task 2

1. B; 2. B; 3. A; 4. B; 5. D; 6. D; 7. A; 8. B; 9. A; 10. C

Supplementary Reading

1. F；2. F；3. T；4. T；5. F

Vocabulary Tips

1. pharmacology；2. prescribe；3. pharmacist；4. Pharmacopoeia；5. describe

Translation for Reference

课文 A

古代药学的发展

史前发展情况

药学随着人类的发展而发展。古人本能地通过观察鸟兽进行学习。最初尝试用清凉的水、树叶、泥土或泥浆来舒缓一些病痛。通过试验，他知道了什么对他最有益。最后，他用自己积累的知识造福他人。虽然这些方法都很粗糙，但今天的许多药物都源于早期人类所能接触到的简单的、基本的药材。

古巴比伦药学的发展

巴比伦是古代美索不达米亚的瑰宝，常被称为文明的摇篮，它（为世界）提供了已知最早的关于药师实践的记录。在当时的时代（约公元前 2600 年）从医者集牧师、药剂师和医生于一身。当今现代医药、医疗和精神护理中都能找到对应的古巴比伦的方法。

中国古代药学的发展

传说中国的药学起源于神农（大约公元前 2000 年），他发现并验证了几百种草药的药用价值。中国世代传颂神农尝百草并著书《本草经》的故事。《本草经》记载了 365 种草药。神农从田野、沼泽和树林中采集了许多草药、树皮和根茎并验证其药理功能，当今的药学还认可这些发现，因此神农被中国的中药行业视为守护神。

《爱柏氏纸草纪事》时代

虽然埃及的医学可以追溯到公元前 2900 年，但公元前 1500 年的《爱柏氏纸草纪事》是最著名、最重要的药用书籍，书中收集 800 个处方，记载 700 种药物。古埃及的制药由两个或两个以上的梯队共同完成，包括药物的采集和制备者，以及"制造主管"或首席药剂师。人们认为他们在"生命之屋"工作。《爱柏氏纸草纪事》可能是由首席药剂师在制药室指导配制药物时口述给抄写员的内容。

泰奥弗拉斯托斯——植物学之父

泰奥弗拉斯托斯（约公元前 300 年）是希腊早期最伟大的哲学家和自然科学家之一，被称为"植物学之父"。他描述了 500 多种植物，并设计了一套先进的植物分类方案。他关于草药的医学性状特性的观察和描述，即使在现有知识下看还是非常准确的。

盖伦——药物配制的实验者

在药学和医学领域中都被人们熟知和尊敬的古代人物中，盖伦无疑是最重要的一员。盖伦（公元 129—210 年）在罗马从事并教授药学和医学；他的药物制备和复方原则统治了西方世界 1500 年；他的名字至今仍与用机械方法配制的一类制剂联系在一起——盖仑制剂（或传统草本制剂）。盖伦是冷霜配方的创始人，与今天所知的配方基本相似。盖伦发明的许多制药方法在当今现代配药实验室中也还有沿用。

课文 B

药剂师

药剂师向患者分发处方药，并提供安全使用处方药的专业知识。他们还可能进行健康检查，提供免疫接种，监督病人的药物治疗，并就健康的生活方式提供建议。

药剂师类型

社区药剂师在零售药店工作，如连锁药店或独立拥有的药店。他们给病人分发药物，并回答病人关于处方、非处方药或其可能存在的任何健康问题。他们还可能提供一些初级保健服务，如注射流感疫苗。

临床药师在医院、诊所和其他医疗机构工作。他们较少分发药物。相反，他们直接参与病人的护理。临床药师可能会与医生或医疗团队一起在医院查房。他们建议给病人用药，并监督药物的剂量和时间。他们还可能进行一些医学测试，并为病人提供建议。例如，在糖尿病诊所工作的药剂师可能会就如何及何时服药等问题向患者提供咨询、建议健康食物的选择，以及监测患者的血糖。

药剂师顾问就病人用药或改善药房服务向保健机构或保险供应商提供建议。他们也可能直接给病人提供建议，比如帮助老年人管理他们的处方药物。

制药行业药剂师的工作领域包括市场营销、销售或研发。他们可能设计或进行临床药物试验，并帮助开发新药。他们还可能帮助建立安全法规，确保药品的质量控制。

有些药剂师是大学教授。他们可以教药学专业的学生或进行研究。

药剂师应具备的重要素质

分析能力。药剂师必须有效地提供安全的药物。要做到这一点，他们必须能够评估病人的需求和医生的指令，并有广泛的知识，能了解药物效果及在合适的情况给予特定药物。

沟通技能。药剂师经常给病人提供建议。例如，他们可能需要解释如何吃药，以及药的副作用。他们还需要为药学技术人员和实习生提供明确的指导。

计算机技能。药剂师需要掌握计算机技能，以便能使用药剂师组织所采用的任何电子健康记录（EHR）系统。

注重细节。药剂师有责任确保他们所给的处方药的准确性。他们必须能够找到需要的信息来决定什么药物适合什么样的病人，因为不正确的使用药物会造成严重的健康风险。

管理技能。药剂师——尤其是那些经营零售药店的药剂师——必须具备良好的管理技能，包括管理库存和监管员工的能力。

药剂师的教育培养

未来的药师必须具有药学博士学位（Pharm. D）。药学博士课程包括化学、药理学和医学伦理学。学生们还可以在医院和零售药店等不同的环境中完成有监督的工作经历，有时称为实习。

一些拥有自己药房的药剂师可能在获得药学博士学位以外，会选择获得工商管理硕士学位。其他人可能会获得公共卫生学位。

药剂师还必须在整个职业生涯中接受继续教育课程，以跟上药学的最新进展。

补充阅读

医院药剂师在患者护理中的作用不断扩大

肯·克里兹纳

2019 年 5 月 23 日

为什么医院的药剂师在患者护理中扮演着越来越重要的角色，为什么他们的参与可以提高药物治疗效果并减少错误。

医院药剂师与其他执业环境中的药剂师并无不同。他们的主要目标是确保患者可以安全使用药物。

但是，除此目的之外，医院药师（也称为卫生系统或临床药师）的作用涵盖了广泛的职责，其最终目标是在住院期间提供优质的护理，确保护理的无缝过渡并减少用药错误的数量。

医院药剂师会就诊断进行咨询，检查患者图表，进行患者评估以推荐治疗方案，并选择合适的药物剂量并评估其有效性。

"在卫生系统中，药剂师比以往任何时候都更多地直接参与患者护理"佛罗里达州墨尔本市临床顾问药剂师诺曼·托马克说，"药剂师有令人难以置信的机会来改善患者的治疗效果。我看到这种情况越来越多。"

随着基于价值的支付模式的持续趋势，医院药剂师正在积极参与降低再入院率的工作。

"在医院中，药剂师的角色正在从以分销为中心的模式转变为更多以服务提供为重点"美国卫生系统学会药理实践促进中心主任，药学博士，药剂师埃里克·迈瑞卡说，"他们是跨专业团队的一部分，可能跨越不同的护理环境。部分原因是转向基于价值的护理，例如先天性肌无力综合征（CMS）的质量指标和再入院目标。"

卫生系统如何使用药剂师减少再入院

对于患有慢性疾病的病人，医院药剂师可以与医生合作管理疾病状态，例如高血压和慢性阻塞性肺疾病，主要是通过病人教育和咨询，药物安全管理，药物审查，监测与和解，特定风险因素的检测、控制和结果等方式。

这些互动的例子表明，医院药剂师作为护理团队的一部分参与的价值。

"很多时候，有些在医院工作的药剂师身体会承受压力"美国药剂师协会（APhA）的女发言人，医学博士布鲁克·戴维·里维埃斯说，"在家有用的东西在医院可能就没用了。医院的药剂师可以确保处方和剂量在临床上是合适的。"

戴维·里维埃斯将医院药剂师描述为监管机构。她指出："我们是安全网。""提供者可以订购药物治疗，但只有在药剂师进行安全检查后才能进行药物治疗。这是药剂师在住院环境中做出的最大贡献。"

更少的用药错误

大量研究表明，医院药剂师通过与其他提供者的协作，为更安全地使用药物作出了实质性贡献，并且他们通过进行监督来改善入院和出院对账的质量（减少的药物差异）。

进一步的研究表明，与护士相比，药剂师发现每位病人服用的药物数量明显增多，包括更多的非处方药和草药，并且他们与病人的门诊药房接触的频率明显高于护士。

根据 2016 年 3 月发表的一项研究，当药剂师而不是医生完成住院期间的患者药物核对时，错误更少。

"有很多研究记录了医院药剂师的重要作用"博特强调说。

（肯·克里兹纳是俄亥俄州克利夫兰市的自由作家）

Unit 3

Keys to Exercises

Warming-up

1. D；2. B；3. C；4. A

Reading A

Task 1

1. The drugs are available for use in the diagnosis, cure, treatment, or prevention of disease.

2. Prescription drugs are medications that require a prescription, from a doctor or other medical professional authorized to write prescriptions, to be dispensed. Over-the-counter drugs are medications consumers can purchase without a prescription at drug stores, groceries, or other stores.

3. In the U. S. , several types of medical professionals can write prescriptions, including physicians, physician assistants, dentists, optometrists, nurse practitioners, psychiatrists, and some advanced practice nurses.

4. Because prescription medications are specially tailored for use by a specific person for a specific use.

5. The biggest difference is that prescription medications require a doctor or other medical professional's authorization to obtain. And they differ in purpose, target, potency, dosage and price.

Task 2

1. g；2. a；3. b；4. h；5. f；6. c；7. e；8. i；9. d；10. j

Task 3

1. to diagnose；2. regarding；3. authorization；4. intended；5. interacting

Task 4

1. There are a variety of drugs available for use in the diagnosis, cure, treatment, or prevention of disease.

2. OTC medications are considered safe for just about everyone and may have a variety of intended purposes.

3. Whether you're taking prescription or non-prescription medication, it's important that you follow the directions and use the medication only for its intended purpose.

4. In most cases, a prescription medication will be far more expensive than an OTC drug.

5. Keeping up with expiration dates will also help you avoid taking ineffective drugs.

Listening & Speaking

Task 1

Overseas Students in China: Chinese Medicine

David: I understand that Chinese medicine is based more on natural products while western medicine more on chemical products. Are Chinese people more accustomed to Chinese medicine?

Liu Yang: It's hard to say. For example, for certain chronic diseases, Chinese traditional medicine is better than western medicine.

David: What other differences are there between Chinese and western medicine?

Liu: Since Traditional Chinese Medicine believes that the different parts of the human body are all interrelated, it strives to bring balance to the body as a whole. In contrast, Western Medicine considers the human body as a machine made up of individual and independent parts.

David: It sounds like Chinese medicine is more wholesome than western medicine. However, 70% of the medicine is western medicine. Why do people buy western medicine instead of Chinese medicine?

Liu: As I mentioned earlier, Chinese medicine is more effective for specific diseases. Chinese medicine does not represent the whole pharmaceutical market, only about 20%-25% of it. There are certain categories of pharmaceuticals such as antibiotics that are not included in Chinese medicine.

David: But antibiotics can be harmful if they are taken too often. All in all, Chinese medicine sounds healthier. Maybe I should go see a Chinese doctor if I get sick. Thanks.

1. F; 2. F; 3. T; 4. T; 5. F

Task 2

I Need to Refill This Prescription

Patient: Excuse me. I need to refill this prescription.

Pharmacist: It says on the bottle here that you can have two refills.

Patient: Yes, I need to refill it today.

Pharmacist: Alright. ⋯ (After a short while.) I'm sorry, Miss, according to our file, this prescription has already been refilled twice.

Patient: I was worried about that. I couldn't remember if I had it refilled twice yet or not.

Pharmacist: Well, it looks like you have. You will need to see your doctor to get a new prescription.

Patient: Listen. This is an emergency. I tried to call my doctor, but he is out of town. So, I can't see him in time. I need this medicine. It is for skin condition. I've run out. Can you just refill it once more?

Pharmacist: I'm sorry, Miss. We can't do it. We must follow the prescription. And this prescription has run out.

Patient: But I need it. Please. Refill it for me just this once. I can go to the doctor around ten days from now. Then I'll have another prescription.

Pharmacist: Miss, I understand your problem. But it is against the law for us to sell certain medicines without a prescription. It's the law. I can't do anything about it. I'm sorry. We never sell medicine unless we have a proper prescription. Never.

Patient: But I have a prescription. I just need more of it.

Pharmacist: A prescription must be valid. It cannot be an expired prescription. I'm sorry, Miss. It's the law. You will have to find another doctor who will prescribe this for you.

Patient: Oh, it will be so expensive! I have a special medical plan, and I can only see one doctor. It will cost me a lot of money to see another doctor.

Pharmacist: Miss, I just can't help you on this. I know it is frustrating when this happens. But there is nothing I can do about it. I'm so sorry.

1. B; 2. B; 3. C; 4. C; 5. D

Task 3

Pharmacy-Health-Prescription

I recently graduated from a pharmacy school. Now I work as a staff pharmacist in a local drug store. My <u>supervisor</u> has a Doctor of Pharmacy degree. He <u>oversees</u> the entire operation. Although it is a rather small pharmacy, we do carry most of the prescription drugs on a daily basis. In case the <u>prescribed</u> drugs are not available in stock; I can usually place an order for them in less than 24 hours. Most of our clients are senior citizens. Some of them come in quite frequently, and the most prescribed drug is the <u>painkiller</u>. I have learned how to file prescription insurance claims, divide drugs into small packages, and locate the right direction labels for the pills. I take my job very <u>seriously</u> because it directly affects people's health. A responsible attitude is a must because any careless mistakes can lead to grave consequences.

    1. supervisor; 2. oversees; 3. prescribed; 4. painkiller; 5. seriously

Reading B

Task 1

1. C; 2. D; 3. B; 4. A; 5. D

Task 2

1. 从生物学角度来说，药物主要作用于我们的大脑，改变我们的情绪和身体的生理状况。
2. 根据定义，药物是进入生命系统后影响或改变生理功能的化学物质。
3. 例如，止痛药减轻疼痛，而消炎药减轻身体的炎症。
4. 不同的药物有不同的作用，也就是说，每种药物都有其自己的反应方式被称为药物作用。
5. 这种药物分类在临床试验中更有帮助。

Practical Writing

Resume

Name: Liu Yang   Sex: Male   Date of Birth: May 12th, 1992

Address: No. 65, Donghai Road, Nanfang

Mobile: 15312345678   E-mail: liuyang@ qq. com

Position Applied for: Pharmaceutical Sales Executive

Educational Background:

Sept. 2009-July 2012: Studied in Jiangnan Vocational College, majoring in Pharmacy.

Won scholarships (during 2010-2011 academic years).

Obtained the certificate of the computer test in 2011.

Sept. 2006-July 2009: Studied in No. 1 High School of Nanfang.

Work Experience:

July 2012-now: Working in ABC Company, responsible for drug sales and management.

Be familiar with office work and skilled at using computers.

Received technical training both at home and abroad during the working period.

Strong Points: Be good at communications and able to cooperate well with teammates.

Hobbies: Football and Photographing

Grammar Tips

Task 1

1. S + V + O; 2. S + V + IO + DO; 3. S + V + O + OC; 4. S + V; 5. S + V + P;

6. S + V + P; 7. S + V + IO + DO; 8. S + V + P; 9. S + V; 10. S + V + O + OC

Task 2

1. A; 2. A; 3. A; 4. A; 5. C; 6. B; 7. B; 8. A; 9. D; 10. A

Supplementary Reading

1. F; 2. F; 3. T; 4. F; 5. T

Vocabulary Tips

1. Optics; 2. allergen; 3. optical; 4. allopathic; 5. hypersensitive

Translation for Reference

课文 A

处方药和非处方药：您知道区别吗?

药物是一种化学物质，它通过与生物系统相互作用而产生某些变化。有各种各样的药物可用来诊断、治愈、治疗或预防疾病。这些药物分为两大类：处方药和非处方药。

处方药和非处方药在改善世界各地患者的健康和保健方面各有其作用。了解处方药和非处方药之间的区别，可以帮助患者在当地药店和从药品批发商那里购买药品时做出更好的用药决定。

在美国，食品和药物管理局决定哪些药物需要药店开出处方。可以开具处方的医疗专业人员有以下几种类型，医生、医师助理、牙医、验光师、执业护士、精神病医生和一些高级执业护士。兽医只能给动物开处方。

在中国和许多其他国家，处方药是指需要医生或其他有资格开具处方的医疗专业人员开具处方才能配药的药物。非处方药是指消费者无需处方就可以在药店、杂货店或其他商店购买的药物。

关键的不同点

当然，处方药和非处方药最大的区别在于，处方药需要医生或其他医疗专业人士的授权才能获得。以下是处方药和非处方药的一些主要区别：

处方药是专门为特定的人针对特定的用途而定制的。非处方药被认为对几乎每个人都是安全的，其可能有各种各样的预期目的。当医生开处方时，他们会考虑病人的很多信息，包括他们目前的状况，他们可能服用的其他药物，他们的生命体征值，以及他们可能有的药物过敏。这就是为什么对一个人安全有效的处方药对另一个人可能是危险的。

非处方药只能用于治疗小病。重大疾病需要使用更强效的处方药和其他医疗手段。

非处方药的药效不如处方药，但它们的安全系数更大。这意味着更多的人可以安全地使用非处方药，而不是使用专门定制的处方药。

非处方药的剂量通常比处方药低。有相当多的处方药可以用作非处方药，因为在非处方药销售时，剂量要比作为处方药的剂量低得多。

一般来说，非处方药比处方药便宜。有些非专利处方药比非处方药便宜，但是，在大多数情况下，处方药要比非处方药贵得多。用于治疗癌症和其他严重疾病的药物，处方药的价格可能非常昂贵。

无论你是在服用处方药还是非处方药，重要的是按照说明用药，并且只用于药物的预期用途。保持药物在有效期内还能帮助你避免服用无效药物。

课文 B

药物的分类

药物介绍

药物，这个词对我们来说并不陌生。然而，这个词通常会引起很多人的反感。到目前为止，我们听说药物是上瘾的物质，是被宠坏的一代的原因。这主要是因为人们一直在滥用药物导致死亡，甚至是受欢迎的人的死亡。

是的，它们会让人上瘾，但你知道吗，它们都是无害的。从生物学角度来说，药物主要作用于我们的大脑，改变我们的情绪和身体的生理状况。然而，由于有各种各样的药物，包括合法的和非法的，后者造成了大多数的问题。

话虽如此，在这一章我们将主要讨论合法药物及其分类。

药物是什么？

根据定义，药物是进入生命系统后影响或改变生理功能的化学物质。它们可以是天然的，也可以是合成的。

化学上，它们是低原子质量和分子质量结构。当一种药物具有治疗活性并用于疾病的诊断、治疗或预防时，它被称为药物（合法药物）。它们以体内的大分子为目标，并产生生物反应。它们中的大多数会中断神经系统（尤其是大脑），以产生适当的生物反应。然而，它们在高剂量下可能是有毒的，这个剂量通常被称为致死剂量。

药物分类

药物分类可以在一定标准的基础上进行。下面列出了一些药物分类方法。

（1）基于药理效应的药物分类

药物是如何影响有机体的细胞被称为药理效应。不同类型的药物对生物体有不同的药理效应。例如，止痛药减轻疼痛，而消炎药减轻身体的炎症。因此，药物可以根据药理效应进行分类。

（2）基于药物作用反应的药物分类

不同的药物有不同的作用，也就是说，每种药物都有其自己的反应方式（药物作用）。根据药物如何产生反应，其作用更加具体。例如，治疗高血压的药物很多，但每种药物都有不同的药物作用。所有的高血压药物降低血压的途径不同。

（3）基于化学结构的药物分类

这是一种常见的药物分类方法。一般来说，具有相同药物作用和药理效应的药物具有基本相同的骨架结构和分支的细微变化。这就是为什么有些药物比另一些更有潜力。例如，所有的磺胺类化合物都有相同的骨架结构。

（4）基于分子靶点的药物分类

药物以体内的大分子为靶点，产生生物反应。这种大分子称为靶分子或药物靶。具有相同作用机制的药物会有相同的靶点。这种药物分类在临床试验中更有帮助。

补充阅读

了解中西医，以达到最大的治疗效益

曹传海，布朗 B.

南佛罗里达大学药学院药理学学系

美国坦帕市布鲁斯唐斯大道 12901 号邮编：33612

药物可以追溯到人类的起源，因为食物和药物是相互交织的。有些食物可以药用，有些具有药用价值的食物也可作为日常食物使用。草药也是如此。

当我们走向工业化，现代西医成为主要的医学实践。从此，草药在疾病治疗中逐渐失去了主导地位。我们面临着选择使用传统医学还是现代医学的挑战。传统医学也被称为传统中医，包括外科、艾灸、火罐、针灸、按摩、草药和营养医学。现代医学，即西医，包括外科手术和最常见的单分子药物。

中西医的主要区别

中医通过病人的症状和外表（眼睛、皮肤、舌色和脉搏）进行诊断，然后寻求解决整个问题，重点是防止任何潜在的不良影响。

西医治疗症状，把目标或目标器官看作是与身体其他部分分离的，而不是作为一个相互联系的整体。

西医通过实验室检测进行诊断，侧重于消除症状，但通常不能解决对身体的不良影响。

中医注重对身体整体的治疗，并认识到身体是一个相互联系的生物系统。治疗改变身体的整体状况，包括免疫系统，但也照顾特定的目标问题。

药物起效时间

西药一般具有快速起效或立竿见影的效果，所以对威胁生命的疾病非常有效。然而，与这些药物相关的主要问题是，即使这是拯救生命的方法，它们也可能会对身体其他部位造成潜在的损害。

中药的目的是预防不良反应和治疗疾病。药物起效的时间较西药长，但考虑到潜在的不良反应，使用更安全。它还可以预防由西药治疗引起的继发性疾病或后遗症。

中西结合，治疗效果最大化

传统医学中有一种原理叫做"君臣佐使"，它包括四种功能：

1. 君药：直接对抗或攻击与疾病相关的病理的药物或分子。

2. 臣药：能增强药物功能的药物或分子。

3. 佐药：可以防止君药的副作用，以限制异常反应。

4. 使药：能把君药功能带到靶点的药物或分子。

使用哪种方法治疗疾病本身并没有好坏之分。我们认为，治疗人类疾病的最佳方法应该遵循中医"君臣佐使"的原则。以西药缓解当前症状，以中药并举解决疾病根源、预防疾病复发的一种综合疗法。这种方法以西药为主要元素，而中药则作为一种"辅助传话者"和"信使"。

Unit 4

Keys to Exercises

Warming-up

1. B；2. A；3. D；4. C

Reading A

Task 1

1. Chinese materia medica refers to the botanical, mineral, and zoological substances applied by traditional Chinese medicine as a primary weapon for preventing and treating diseases.

2. No. Some medical substances are either from other parts of the world or have been introduced and planted in China.

3. About 2000 years ago.

4. It mainly expounds the basic knowledge of Chinese medicine in terms of source, nature, processing, actions, indications, as well as its basic theories and administration. .

5. Preventing and treating cardiovascular diseases.

Task 2

1. g；2. c；3. d；4. e；5. f；6. b；7. h；8. i；9. j；10. a

Task 3

1. treatment；2. indication；3. medicinal；4. natural；5. action

Task 4

1. Some people are of the wrong impression that Chinese materia medica are all produced in China.

2. Chinese material medica has been used as a primary weapon for preventing and treating diseases.

3. Chinese people have accumulated rich medical experiences.

4. Science of Chinese Materia Medica plays an essential role in the historical development of traditional Chinese medicine.

5. Yín Xìng Yè is known for its excellent actions of preventing and treating cardiovascular disease.

Listening & Speaking

Task 1

Could You Fill the Prescription for Me?

David：This is my prescription. Could you fill it for me, please?

Chemist：Certainly.

David：Thank you.

Chemist：You're welcome. Well, let me see. It will take about five minutes.

David：OK.

Chemist: All right. This is your herbal medicine.

David: Could you tell me what I should do with it?

Chemist: Every morning leave one packet to soak in 500ml of cold water for one hour and a half. Then use strong fire to boil it up, and cook over slow fire for 30 minutes. Turn off the heat, leave it to cool and pour the liquid into a cup for drinking. Do not let any of the leaves go into the cup.

David: It is quite complicated. By the way, can I use a steel pan?

Chemist: No, you can't do that. You'd better use an earthenware pot.

David: Thank you very much. I've learnt a lot from you today.

Chemist: You're welcome. I hope you will recover in no time.

1. T; 2. F; 3. F; 4. F; 5. T

Task 2

Cordyceps

Leo: My, it looks too queer.

Tom: So it is. It is called cordyceps, a tonic only available in China. Many ancient Chinese medicine journals have recorded that it can cure such ailments as night sweat, pain at waist and knees , and anaemia. Besides, it has no side effect.

Leo: Great! Would you please tell me how to take it?

Tom: Certainly. Fill 3 or 5 pieces of cordyceps in to a cleaned duck and cook with the whole duck, or stew it with chicken.

Leo: That sounds very interesting

Tom: Please don't take turnip and garlic when taking cordyceps.

Leo: Thank you very much.

1. C; 2. B; 3. D; 4. A; 5. C

Task 3

Jinhua Qinggan Granule was developed during the 2009 H1N1 influenza <u>pandemic</u>. It consists of 12 herbal components including honeysuckle, mint and licorice and can <u>clear</u> heat and detoxify lungs. It has a curative effect in treating <u>mild</u> and moderate patients and can also improve the <u>recovery rate</u> of lymphocyte and white blood cells as well as reduce the rate of patients turning more severe. A comparative experiment showed that patients who took Jinhua Qinggan Granule tested <u>negative</u> for coronavirus two and a half days earlier than a group that did not take the granule. The group treated with the granule also took eight days to show improvement, while the other group took 10. 3 days.

1. pandemic; 2. clear; 3. mild ; 4. recovery rate; 5. negative

Reading B

Task 1

1. A; 2. B; 3. D; 4. C; 5. B

Task 2

1. 在新冠病毒尚未攻克之际，中医药再次成为争论的焦点。

2. 虽然一副中成药已被证明能有效治疗轻症患者，但西方医学界对此仍持怀疑态度，以缺乏严格的实验数据为理由，质疑中药的临床疗效。

3. 面对这种让世界猝不及防的新病毒，大国都在科学前沿奋战，在缺乏广泛认可的疫苗的情况下，制定临床方案。

4. 西医是建立在药理学和毒理学的基础上的，而中医则是建立在几千年的经验基础上的。

5. 中药，特别是在预防和治疗慢性病方面，有其独特性和优势。随着人口老龄化成为大趋势，中药将会更适合这类人群。

Practical Writing

Shijiazhuang Yiling Pharmaceutical Co., Ltd., a national key high-tech enterprise, was founded by Wu Yiling, Academician of the Chinese Academy of Engineering. Under his leadership, Yiling Pharmaceutical has always adhered to the development strategy of taking the technology innovation as the guide and taking the market as the lead. Therefore, the five-in-one unique operating model, "Theory, Clinical Practices, Scientific Research, Industry, Education", has been established and a new drug development and innovation technology system guided by theoretical innovation of traditional Chinese medicine collateral disease has been set up. The five-in-one unique operating model got highly recognition of the leaders of the Ministry of Science and Technology of PRC, appreciating it as "the pioneering work in the industrialization of scientific and technological achievements in TCM".

Grammar Tips

Task 1

1. 主语从句；2. 表语从句；3. 主语从句；4. 表语从句；5. 宾语从句；6. 宾语从句；7. 表语从句；8. 宾语从句；9. 宾语从句；10. 主语从句

Task 2

1. C；2. D；3. C；4. B；5. A；6. C；7. A；8. B；9. B；10. D

Supplementary Reading

1. F；2. T；3. T；4. F；5. T

Vocabulary Tips

1. cardiac；2. panorama；3. electrocardiogram；4. toxicity；5. panacea

Translation for Reference

课文 A

中药和中药学

中药包括植物药、动物药以及矿物药，是中医预防、治疗疾病的主要手段。

一些人误认为中药都产自中国。但实际上，一些中药产自国外；一些中药是从国外引进、在国内种植的。

在早期的历史中，当人们依靠采集植物和狩猎动物作为主要的食物来源时，逐渐认识到这些植物或动物对人体具有有益或有害的影响，这就是中药的起源。中国悠久的文明史可以追溯到6000年前。中国人口众多，幅员辽阔，资源丰富。中国人在生存和疾病防治方面积累了丰富的医学经验，逐渐形成了中药的理论体系。早在2000多年前，《黄帝内经》和《神农本草经》的编撰就已经形成了较为完整的中药理论体系：前者（《黄帝内经》）系统表述了中药学相关理论及其应用原则，如四性五味、五脏与性味的关系、五脏疾病的药物选择等；后者（《神农本草经》）则详细描述了365种草药的性味、作用及适应证。

作为中医药的基础学科，中药学主要介绍了中药的基础理论和施用，还介绍了中药的来源、性状、炮制、作用、适应证等方面的基础知识。

在中国古代，中药及其相关著作因其主要成分是中草药而被称为"本草学"。历史上有关中药的书籍种类繁多、新草药不断增加且新用途不断完善，这些都是璀璨的中华文化瑰宝。中国中药资源丰富，中药学内容丰富，中药种类繁多。

中药学取得了巨大成就，不仅在中国及邻国的医药史中发挥了重要作用，而且对世界医药的发展也产生了重要影响。对中药的研究，尤其是对生药的研究，已成为国际医学领域的热点之一。每年都有新产品从中药中被提取出来，例如：银杏叶提取物以其预防和治疗心血管疾病的功效而闻名。欧洲制药企业因此获得了巨额利润。

课文 B

让中医药走向世界

全球医学界就中医药的疗效争论了几十年。在新冠病毒尚未攻克之际，中医药再次成为争论的焦点。虽然中成药已被证明能有效治疗轻症患者，但西方医学界对此仍持怀疑态度，以缺乏严格的实验数据为理由，质疑中药的临床疗效。

面对这种让世界猝不及防的新病毒，大国都在科学前沿奋战，在缺乏广泛认可的疫苗的情况下，制定临床方案。在中国提出的345个治疗方案中，中医药治疗方案占111个。

就像过去一样，"历史经验"再次受到审视。将中药推向全球市场的首次尝试要追溯到1997年，当时用于治疗冠心病的"复方丹参滴丸"的制造商获得了美国食品和药物管理局（FDA）的批准。此后，有10多种中成药进行了尝试，但最终只有3种进入Ⅲ期临床试验。这三种药分别是复方丹参滴丸、穿心莲提取物和血脂康。

FDA于2004年发布了一份行业植物药物开发指南草案，并于2016年定稿。指南指出，由于植物药物可能仍然是复杂的混合物，"植物药物中的活性成分的提纯和鉴定都是可选的，而不是必需的。"它还指出，人类广泛使用植物产品的临床信息可用于新药研发和监管审查。

西医是建立在药理学和毒理学的基础上，而中医则是建立在几千年经验的基础上。中草药具有复杂的化学成分，因此需要潜心研究其有效成分，以及这些成分之间是如何相互作用来缓解某些症状的。

要增强中医在全球的影响力，最重要的因素是强大的科学性、共识、质量和对相关临床研究的投入。了解中药的好处，并将其与西方疗法结合起来使用，是提高全球草药接受度的关键。随着新冠肺炎疫情的全面爆发，中西医结合的用药效果非常好，但是建立药物产品背后的科学是非常重要的，更多关于疗效的数据，正在生成。

新冠肺炎激发了西方国家对中医药的兴趣，但中医药要在世界范围内推广仍存在困难。人们对中医的广泛认可度并不那么乐观，但至少人们已经开始认识到：中医可以治疗大流行病中的急性病毒感染。我国在中药种植和销售规范方面取得了长足的进步，目前相关产品的合格率已达到80%以上。需要做的还有很多。

中药，将会发挥越来越重要的作用。中药，特别是在预防和治疗慢性病方面，有其独特性和优势。随着人口老龄化成为大趋势，中药将会更适合这类人群。

中医药必将走向国际化，这只是个时间问题。

补充阅读

连花清瘟

连花清瘟是一种常见的用于治疗普通感冒和流感的中药。它由13种中药组成，对轻症和普通患者有疗效，尤其在缓解发热、咳嗽和疲劳方面，疗效显著。它可降低病情恶化的发生率，患者用药后，病毒转阴。

2020年4月14日，以岭药业宣布，以岭药业及其子公司北京以岭药业已收到国家药监局关于连花清瘟胶囊、连花清瘟颗粒新适应证申请的批准文件。连花清瘟胶囊（颗粒）新增新冠肺炎适应证申请获批。其可用于新冠肺炎轻症患者的治疗，常见症状有发热、咳嗽和疲劳，用法用量增至7~10天。

连花清瘟胶囊（颗粒）成为中国治疗新冠肺炎最常推荐的中成药。国家卫生健康委员会和国家中医药管理局发布的第四到第七版新冠肺炎诊疗方案，建议采用中成药连花清瘟胶囊（颗粒）帮助在医学观察期间的患者预防和治疗疾病。

连花清瘟胶囊（颗粒）治疗新冠肺炎的疗效已通过基础实验和临床研究的证实。钟南山团队最近在国际期刊《药理学研究》上发表了一篇题为《连花清瘟对新型冠状病毒具有抗病毒、抗炎作用》的论文，这是首篇关于中成药治疗SARS-CoV-2的基础研究文章。本研究发现连花清瘟能明显抑制新型冠状病毒在细胞内的复制，患者服用后，细胞内病毒粒子的表达水平明显降低。

据报道，该批准是在原有批准的适应证的基础上增加的"新冠肺炎轻型，普通型"的新适应证。与此同时，新批处方药规范并没有否定原有的非处方药定位。

截至目前，连花清瘟胶囊已在中国香港特别行政区、中国澳门特别行政区、巴西、印度尼西亚、加拿大、莫桑比克、罗马尼亚等地注册为"中成药""药""植物药"和"天然保健品"，并已获准上市销售。

Unit 5

Keys to Exercises

Warming-up

1. D; 2. A; 3. B; 4. C

Reading A

Task 1

1. Discovery and Development, Preclinical Research, Clinical Research, FDA Review, FDA Post-Market Safety Monitoring.

2. Funding comes from several areas including government, grants, and revenues.

3. Preclinical research is involved in testing the drug on animals and basic testing for safety flags.

4. If a drug is cleared from preclinical trials, it moves on to clinical testing which involves human trials.

5. If a submission is accepted, the FDA will provide a response within 6 to 10 months.

Task 2

1. e; 2. i; 3. h; 4. c; 5. g; 6. b; 7. a; 8. j; 9. d; 10. f

Task 3

1. mandated; 2. testing; 3. cleared; 4. followed; 5. monitoring

Task 4

1. Each drug begins with discovery and development in a lab.

2. Clinical trials follow a typical series from early, small-scale, phase 1 studies to late-stage, large scale, phase 3 studies.

3. The Food and Drug Administration is one of the primary regulators involved in all aspects of the drug market.

4. If a submission is accepted, the FDA will provide a response within 6 to 10 months.

5. The FDA monitors all types of drug advertising for accuracy.

Listening & Speaking

Task 1

Which is One of the Most Powerful Killers of Bacteria?

Leo: Tom, do you think which is one of the most powerful killers of bacteria?

Tom: Penicillin, definitely. It has saved lives and prevented suffering all over the world. But it was discovered quite by accident.

Leo: By accident? Can you tell me the story?

Tom: Of course, In 1928, Dr. Alexander Fleming was looking for something that would kill bacteria. One evening he failed to place a cover on one of the plates, when he came the next morning he saw some blue-green mould had grown during the night. But around the outside of the uncovered plate the bacteria were still flourishing while in the area close to the mould there were none. They had somehow disappeared. Fleming put some of the mould together with more bacteria of the same kind, the germs were also destroyed. He seemed to have discovered a powerful antibiotic.

Leo: Excellent, so if Fleming had not noticed that small area of mould on his plate, he would not have discovered this powerful antibiotic.

Tom: Yeah, but it was not until 1940 that scientists were able to find a way of producing penicillin as a powder with an unchanging character.

Leo: So from then, it has been used widely?

Tom: No, it was reported a safe drug for use on humans and made available to doctors until 1941. If Fleming had not discovered penicillin, the antibiotic industry would not have developed so quickly.

Leo: Brilliant, so people value Fleming's work greatly.

1. F; 2. T; 3. F; 4. T; 5. F

Task 2

What is Critical for Commercial Success in Drug Development?

Li Jing: Good afternoon, Professor Chen, thanks for your excellent speech, but I still have some questions. Can you explain what is drug development exactly?

Professor Chen: Drug development comprises all the activities involved in transforming a compound from drug candidate to a product approved for marketing by the appropriate regulatory authorities. Here the drug candidate means the end-product of the discovery phase.

Li Jing: OK, I've got it, thanks. And just now, you have mentioned that efficiency in drug development is critical for commercial success, why?

Professor Chen: You know, drug development accounts for about two-thirds of the total R&D costs. The cost per project is very much greater in the development phase, and increases sharply as the project moves into the later phases of clinical development. So keeping these costs under control is a major concern for management.

Li Jing: I agree, failure of a compound late in development represents a lot of money wasted.

Professor Chen: Yes, you are right. And speed in development is also an important factor in determining sales revenue, as time spent in development detracts from the period of patent protection once the drug goes to market.

Li Jing: Yeah, you mean that as soon as the patent expires, generic competition sharply reduces sales revenue.

Professor Chen: Brilliant! You've got what I have taught today.

Li Jing: Thanks, Professor Chen.

1. A; 2. C; 3. D; 4. B; 5. C

Task 3

Technology is enabling new methods of exploring vaccine candidates for trial, but there are already a few tried and tested ways to make them. In all of them, scientists try to stimulate the body's <u>immune</u> system to combat <u>invasive</u> pathogen. That's commonly done by creating something so similar to the pathogen that the body begins to create <u>antibodies</u> to fight off the real thing. The most common way of doing this is to make what's called <u>attenuated</u> vaccines——those that are made of weaker strains of the actual pathogen. Reared on animal cells outside of human bodies, they are then extracted and <u>injected</u> in a single tiny dose. Vaccines for measles and tuberculosis are created in this way.

1. immune; 2. invasive; 3. antibodies; 4. attenuated; 5. injected

Reading B

Task 1

1. D; 2. D; 3. B; 4. A; 5. C

Task 2

1. 在这项研究的第一阶段，她的小组调查了 2000 多种中药制剂，并确定了 640 种可能具有抗疟活性的配方。

2. 屠呦呦出色地改进了提取技术，使其在低温下进行，而不是像传统的用加热方法。

3. 屠呦呦能够将提取物分成不含抗疟活性的酸性部分，显示出降低毒性和提高抗疟活性的中性部分。

4. 几千年来，恶性疟原虫一直是一种危及生命的疾病，每年仍在世界许多地区，特别是在非洲，威胁着数百万人的生命。

5. 青蒿素的发现被公认为人类征服疟疾之旅的一个重要里程碑。

Practical Writing

> *Join Our Medical English Corner*
>
> <u>Do you want to improve your Medical English?</u>
>
> Come and join us!
>
> Here you can
>
> talk to foreign medical professionals
>
> <u>attend medical lectures</u>
>
> <u>read medical magazines and books</u>
>
> make new friends
>
> <u>share your idea with others</u>
>
> From 6:00 p.m. to 8:00 p.m.
>
> Tuesday, Oct. 13th, 2020
>
> English Park
>
> 13974810582
>
> Students' Union
>
> Oct. 10th, 2020

Grammar Tips

Task 1

1. that；2. which；3. whose；4. who；5. that；6. when；7. where；8. whose；9. which；10. that

Task 2

1. D；2. B；3. D；4. B；5. B；6. D；7. B；8. B；9. A；10. B

Supplementary Reading

1. T；2. F；3. F；4. T；5. F

Vocabulary Tips

1. anti-ageing；2. paramedical；3. parasite；4. antibacterial；5. antibody

Translation for Reference

课文 A

药物研发过程

在整个制药行业，药品在最终销售上市之前，必须经过若干法定流程。对于药物整体来说，最重要的阶段之一是得到美国食品和药物管理局（FDA）的批准。因此，本文介绍了 FDA 为成功开发药物过程勾勒出的五个综合阶段，其中第四个阶段是 FDA 的审查。

第一步：发现和开发

每种药物都是从实验室的发现和开发开始。制药公司花费数百万美元进行研发，包括科学研究和开发药物以进行新的创新。资金可能来自多个领域，包括政府、赠款和财政收入。

第二步：临床前研究

一旦一种药物被发现，它必须经过临床前和临床研究，并有与审查过程相关的支持报告。临床前研究是一个基本的初步阶段，涉及在动物身上测试药物和进行安全标志的基本测试。通常，临床前研究规模不是很大。然而，这些研究必须提供有关剂量和毒性水平的详细信息。在临床前测试之后，研究人员回顾他们的发现，并决定是否应该在人体测试这种药物。

第三步：临床研究

临床研究可能是药物开发中最重要的步骤之一。如果一种药物通过了临床前试验，它就会进入涉及人体试验的临床试验。制药公司和 FDA 有具体的临床试验标准，其中包括参与科学测试的专业人员、被检测人员的选择标准、进行临床试验的环境等。临床试验注册也是必须的，整个行业的医药专业人员都要严格遵守。临床试验遵循一系列的研究流程，从早期、小规模、第一阶段研究到晚期、大规模、第三阶段研究。

第四步：FDA 审查

美国食品和药物管理局是药品市场各个方面的主要监管机构之一。美国高标准的药品审批要求通常会导致药物研发测试的前三个阶段要持续大约 10 到 15 年才能获得批准。在第四阶段，公司将有完整文件记载的研究和发现提交 FDA 审查。如果申请被接受，FDA 将在 6 到 10 个月内给出答复。

第五步：FDA 上市后安全监测

对已上市的药物进行批准后的安全监测有几个方面。FDA 监控所有类型的药物广告的真实性。它还监测与药物相关的投诉和问题。因此，它有权限制药品销售并提出警告。一般来说，FDA 也进行常规的生产检查。此外，FDA 还参与所有药物的专利保护和仿制药过渡。

课文 B

青蒿素：中国的抗疟疾药物

2015 年诺贝尔生理学或医学奖得主之一，屠呦呦，与众多中国科学家一起，发现了青蒿素、蒿甲醚和青蒿琥酯，以及其他青蒿素，将全球抗疟治疗带到了一个新时代，在过去 40 年里拯救了全世界数百万人的生命。

在 20 世纪 60 年代末和 70 年代，屠呦呦是一个抗疟研究小组的负责人，她带领一群年轻学者从中草药中提取和分离出可能具有抗疟活性的成分。在这项研究的第一阶段，她的小组调查了 2000 多种中药制剂，并确定了 640 种可能具有抗疟作用的配方。从大约 200 种中草药中提取出 380 多种提取物，其中包括黄花蒿的提取物，并在啮齿类动物疟疾模型上进行了试验。然而，一开始进展并不顺利，也没有取得显著的成果。

当一种青蒿提取物显示出对寄生虫生长有良好抑制作用时，情况出现了转机，这与东晋葛洪（公元 284—346 年）在《肘后备急方》中记载的青蒿活性一致。屠呦呦出色地改进了提取技术，使其在低温下进行，而不是像传统的用加热方法。她发现最有效的制剂来自黄花蒿的叶子，其对鼠疟原虫有显著抑制作用。屠呦呦能够将提取物分成不含抗疟活性的酸性部分，以及显示出降低毒性和提高抗疟活性的中性部分。

在第一次人体试验之后，屠呦呦和她的团队前往海南验证这种提取物的临床疗效，并在感染了间日疟原虫和恶性疟原虫的病人身上进行了抗疟试验。这些临床试验产生了积极的反馈，与使用氯喹的对照组相比，发热情况好转，血液中的寄生虫迅速消失。屠呦呦接下来研究了黄花蒿的活性成分的分离和纯化。最终，1972 年，她的研究小组成功提取到了一种分子量为 282 Da，分子式为 $C_{15}H_{22}O_5$，熔点为 $156 \sim 157°C$ 的无色结晶体，命名为"青蒿素"。然而，由于当时环境的原因，有关青蒿素的论文发表不多。

几千年来，恶性疟原虫一直是一种危及生命的疾病，每年仍在世界许多地区，特别是在非洲，威胁着数百万人的生命。20 世纪 50 年代，国际社会根除疟疾的努力失败后，疟疾卷土重来。青蒿素是一种新型抗疟剂，其化学结构完全不同，疗效更好，与获得抗药性的传统药物相比，在 20 世纪 80 年代青蒿素及其衍生物在中国治疗数千名疟疾病人的成功引起了全世界的关注。自此，青蒿素的发现被公认为人类征服疟疾之旅的一个重要里程碑。

补充阅读

屠呦呦：中国科学家和植物化学家

屠呦呦（1930 年 12 月 30 日生于中国浙江省宁波市），中国科学家和植物化学家，因分离和研究抗疟物质"青蒿素"而闻名。青蒿素是世界上最有效的抗疟疾药物之一。由于她的发现，屠呦呦获得了 2015 年诺贝尔生理学或医学奖（与爱尔兰出生的美国寄生虫学家威廉·坎贝尔和日本微生物学家大村智共享）。

屠呦呦就读于北京医学院药学系。1955 年获得学位后，她被选入中国中医研究院（后中国中医科学院）。从 1959 年至 1962 年，她参加了原卫生部"全国第三期西医离职学习中医班"。该课程为她以后将中医知识应用于现代药物发现打下了基础。

1967 年，越南战争期间（1955—1975），屠呦呦被任命为"523 项目"负责人。屠呦呦和她的研究团队首先根据民间医学资料和中国古代医学文献中所描述的疗法来鉴定具有抗疟疾活性的植物。她的团队确定了大约 640 种植物和 2000 多种具有潜在抗疟活性的疗法，随后测试了约 200 种植物的 380 种提取物，以发现它们是否有能力从受感染小鼠的血液中清除致疟疾的疟原虫。一种从黄花蒿中提取的青蒿显示出特殊的前景。1971 年，在改进了提取工艺之后，屠呦呦和她的同事们成功地从黄花蒿中分离出了一种无毒的提取物，这种提取物有效地消除了小鼠和猴子身上的疟原虫。此后不久，在疟疾病人中进行了临床研究，发现黄花蒿提取物能迅速控制发热，降低血液中的寄生虫水平。1972 年，屠呦呦及其同事从提取物中分离出活性化合物，并将其命名为青蒿素。

尽管屠呦呦的研究依靠的是古代文献中的信息，但研究中对这种名为"青蒿"的植物的描述甚少，而且她的团队早期试图重现他们对植物抗疟活性的初步发现也失败了。然而，屠呦呦最终发表，并发现青蒿叶中含有青蒿素，这种化合物在相对较低的温度下提取效果最佳。由于当时中国对科学信息的发表有限制，屠呦呦最初被禁止发表她的团队的发现。这一作品最终发表，并在 20 世纪 80 年代初获得了国际观众的广泛好评。21 世纪初，世界卫生组织建议使用以青蒿素为基础的联合药物疗法作为疟疾的一线治疗。

屠呦呦继续研究青蒿素，并开发了第二种抗疟化合物，双氢青蒿素，这是一种生物活性的青蒿素代谢物。2011 年，她因对发现青蒿素作出的贡献而荣获拉斯克－德巴基临床医学研究奖。

Unit 6

Keys to Exercises

Warming-up

1. C；2. B；3. D；4. A

Reading A

Task 1

1. A new drug application is a comprehensive document that must be submitted to the U. S. Food and Drug Administration in order to request approval for marketing a new drug in the United States.

2. NDA document must contain 15 sections.

3. The NDA document must demonstrate the proposed drug's pharmacology, toxicology, and dosage requirements as well as the intended process for manufacturing the drug.

4. The goal of the FDA's Center for Drug Evaluation and Research is to review and act on the priority drug within 6 months after the applications are received.

5. The new drug approval process is excessively onerous, posing a barrier to innovation and causing upward pressure on drug prices.

Task 2

1. f; 2. i; 3. g; 4. b; 5. a; 6. c; 7. d; 8. j; 9. e; 10. h

Task 3

1. priority; 2. be evaluated; 3. sponsored; 4. commercial; 5. innovate

Task 4

1. On the other hand, many have argued that the new drug approval process is excessively onerous, posing a barrier to innovation and causing upward pressure on drug prices.

2. For decades, the regulation and control of new drugs in the United States have been based on the New Drug Application.

3. The document must extensively demonstrate the proposed drug's pharmacology, toxicology, and dosage requirements as well as the intended process for manufacturing the drug.

4. Yet, reaching the NDA stage is far from easy.

5. Once the NDA has been submitted, the likelihood of that drug receiving FDA approval is usually very high.

Listening & Speaking

Task 1

Getting a Prescription Filled

Pharmacist: Good morning. How can I help you?

Patient: Good morning, Please make up this prescription.

Pharmacist: Let me see. Okay, I think we have it. Let me get that for you… here you go.

Patient: Thank you, and can you tell me how I should use it?

Pharmacist: Certainly! You need to take these pills once a day before you go to sleep.

Patient: Okay, how long do I need to take them for?

Pharmacist: Ten days for this one. It's important that you finish all the packages, if you forget to take it at night, you need to take two in the morning.

Patient: Okay, is it safe to take with aspirin?

Pharmacist: No, you can't take aspirin while you are on this, no painkillers allowed.

Patient: I see, are there any side effects?

Pharmacist: Rare but possible drowsiness, dizziness, blurred vision, upset stomach, nervousness, … It is recommended that you avoid physically demanding activities after taking this; also no driving.

Patient: Oh, now I see why I should take it before I go to sleep.

Pharmacist: Exactly!

Patient: Well, okay then. Can I pay with my card?

Pharmacist: Sure! That will be $14. Is there anything else I can help you with?

Patient: No, that would be all, thank you.

Pharmacist: You are welcome, here is your receipt.

Patient: Thank you for your help, have a good day.

Pharmacist: Thank you, you too.

1. F; 2. T; 3. F; 4. T; 5. F

Task 2

Buying Medicine without a Prescription

Patient：I have a terrible cold. Apart from that, have a headache and a cough. Can you suggest something I can take to relieve the symptom?

Pharmacist：Don't you have a prescription?

Patient：No, I haven't gone to see a doctor.

Pharmacist：Are you allergic to any type of medication?

Patient：I don't know exactly. I think that I can take most drugs.

Pharmacist：(picks up a small box) I recommend this brand for quick relief.

Patient：Will this really help?

Pharmacist：According to the label, yes. But if that doesn't help, then drink a cup of hot tea along with some honey. There's no miracle drug to cure a common cold.

Patient：Can you sell me penicillin?

Pharmacist：Sorry, sir. I can't sell it. You must first get a doctor's certificate or prescription.

Patient：Do you have any cough syrup ?

pharmacist：Of course. This is a common medicine.

Patient：That's great.

Pharmacist：Here you are. The instructions on it tell you how to take it. Make sure you read them carefully.

Patient：Thank you for reminding me.

Pharmacist：Anything else?

Patient：No, thank you.

Pharmacist：You're welcome.

1. D；2. C；3. B；4. C；5. D

Task 3

Make sure medication works safely to <u>improve</u> your health, there are 8 drug DOs and DON'Ts for you to follow. DO take each medication <u>exactly</u> as it has been prescribed. DO make sure that all your doctors know about all your medications. DO keep medications out of the reach of children and pets. DON'T change your medication dose or <u>schedule</u> without talking with your doctor. DON'T use medication prescribed for someone else. DON'T crush or break pills unless your doctor <u>instructs</u> you to do so. DON'T use medication that has passed its <u>expiration</u> date. DON'T store your medications in locations that are humid, too hot or too cold.

1. improve；2. exactly；3. schedule；4. instructs；5. expiration

Reading B

Task 1

1. B；2. C；3. D；4. D；5. A

Task 2

1. 为销售进口药品，开发人员必须申请第三类注册途径——进口药品许可证，或第一类注册途径——在中国实施全面开发计划，同时提交新药申请以获得新药批准。

2. 进口药品许可证要求，通过在中国受试者中进行临床试验，来注册新化学实体同时获取所有新的临床适应证。

3. 配对的数量取决于方案、适应证和试验设计，并且必须能为研究提供适当程度的统计学意义。

4. 越来越多的跨国开发人员正在将中国的试验纳入他们的全球项目，使用进口药品许可证这种注册途径接触到大量病人并收集数据，来支持在包括中国在内的多个国家同时进行注册。

5. 一直以来，外国生物制药公司主要担忧的就是中国难以操作的药品审批制度和缓慢的审批流程。

Practical Writing

From： lna@ sina. com
To： sy347@ cam. ac. uk
Subject： New drugs order
Date： 25th October，2020
Dear Sir or Madam，

Thank you for the new drug you recommended. We are very interested in your new drug. We will order 1000 boxes for trying to promote. If the market responses are good, we will increase the quantity. We are wondering if we can have a 5% reduction in price. We look forward to further cooperation in the future.

Yours faithfully，
Zhang Qi

Grammar Tips

1. A；2. C；3. D；4. B；5. A；6. C；7. C；8. D；9. B；10. C；11. B；12. B；13. C；14. D；15. B

Supplementary Reading

1. T；2. F；3. F；4. T；5. T

Vocabulary Tips

1. nausea；2. biocide；3. biochemistry；4. navigate；5. autobiography

Translation for Reference

课文 A

新药申请

几十年来，美国对新药的监管和控制都是以新药申请为基础的。自 1938 年，每一种新药在美国商业化之前都是新药申请批准的实验对象。

什么是新药申请？

新药申请是指为了申请批准在美国销售一种新药，向美国食品和药物管理局提交的一份综合文件，是药物生产商正式向美国食品和药物管理局提出审批的一种新的药物在美国销售和营销的方式。试验性新药在动物研究和人体临床试验阶段收集的数据是新药申请的一部分。

如何申请新药？

进行新药申请是一种新药生命周期里的重要里程碑，受到投资者的密切关注。一旦提交了新药申请，这种药物通过美国食品和药物管理局批准的可能性通常会很高。因此，经常会看到提交新药申请的公司的股价上涨，甚至是在得到美国食品和药物管理局的答复之前。

然而，达到新药申请这个阶段绝非易事。每个新药申请文件必须包含 15 个章节，其中包含详细的实验证据（包括动物和人体研究）。该文件必须广泛地证明所提议的药物的药理学、毒理学和剂量要求，以及制造药物的预期过程。

自从 1938 年通过《食品、药品和化妆品法》以来，新药申请就成为了美国监管和控制新药的基础。从那时起，对《食品、药品和化妆品法》的各种修订逐渐提高了获得批准所需的证据标准。

这些更严格的标准带来的一个后果就是审批过程变得非常耗时。美国食品和药物管理局药物评估和研究中心的目标是，在收到申请的 10 个月内，对至少 90% 的标准药物进行审查，在收到申请后的 6 个月内，对优先药物进行审查。当然，药物研发的整个时间轴往往会延长到 10 年或更长时间。

新药申请的利与弊

制药公司必须要历经多个阶段才能成功的将一种新药推向市场，新药申请过程只是其中之一。从美国食品和药物管理局的角度来看，为了保护公众免受药物损害或误导，这种严格的程序是必要的。另一方面，许多人认为，新药审批流程过于繁琐，对创新构成障碍，对药品价格造成上行压力。

课文 B

进口药品在中国的注册途径

新药是指未曾在中国境内外上市销售的药品。在中国获准上市的药品中，进口药品占很大比例。为销售进口药品，开发人员必须申请第三类注册途径——进口药品许可证，或第一类注册途径——在中国实施全面开发计划，同时提交新药申请以获得新药审批。

在这两种途径的选择中，开发人员需要考虑临床试验申请审查时间的重要性，因为两种途径都需要经过审批的临床试验申请。关键点是该药物在世界其他国家的预期批准时间，因为根据定义，一类药物在进行新药申请时必须没有在任何其他国家获得批准。因此，第三类注册途径是药品进入中国市场最普遍的途径。

进口药品许可证要求，通过在中国受试者中进行临床试验，来注册新化学实体同时获取所有新的临床适应证。通常，在申请第三类进口药品许可证的情况下，要求在中国招募 100 对受试者（即 100 例治疗病人和 300 例生物制剂）进行临床试验，国家药品监督管理局可以对该数字进行灵活调整。配对的数量取决于方案、适应证和试验设计，并且必须能为研究提供适当程度的统计学意义。

国家药品监督管理局关于药物注册的规定，允许在申请进口药品许可证时使用来自一个国际多中心试验的中国数据。越来越多的跨国开发人员正在将中国的试验纳入他们的全球项目，使用进口药品许可证这种注册途径接触到大量病人并收集数据，来支持在包括中国在内的多个国家同时注册。开发人员在实施全球多中心开发项目中，产品在美国和欧洲推出与在中国推出相比，平均要历经四到六年的滞后。这种滞后是因为审批时间上的主要差异而产生的，尤其是对于临床试验申请的审查。

鉴于第三类进口药品许可证的局限性，一些开发人员正在探索另一种选择——以中国全面开发计划为基础追求第一类新药申请。第一类新药申请是国产新药的默认注册途径。根据国家药品监督管理局年度药品注册报告，第一类新药申请批准的数量正在增加。而第一类注册途径要求用

Ⅰ期、Ⅱ期和Ⅲ期的临床试验来证明其安全性和有效性，用于中国新药申请提交和国家药品监督管理局审查。

第一类注册的前三步至少需要两年才能完成。临床试验申请的审批需要近一年，新药申请的审批需要近两年。总时限为 4 到 5 年。对于使用来自全球多中心试验的中国数据，通过第一类途径进行注册，时间可能在美国或者欧盟批准后 12 个月以内，或者在某些情况下，可能会获得全球第一个批准。

一直以来外国生物制药公司主要担忧的是中国难以操作的药品审批制度和缓慢的审批流程。据国家药品监督管理局表示，为加快药品审批进程，中国正在制定缩短批准进口药品上市时间的新措施。

补充阅读

美国的试验性新药

詹姆斯·陈

2018 年 5 月 1 日

在美国，试验性新药是指由制药公司、生物技术公司或其他机构开发并准备在人体上进行临床试验的药物。

试验性新药分为两类：商业新药和研究性新药。这两个类别的最大区别是由谁来申请。正如名称所示，商业新药申请是由想要测试药物并将其推向市场的公司进行的。任何公司都可以申请试验性新药。研究性新药或非商业新药申请是研究人员要求对现有药物进行测试的步骤。当研究人员想要测试已经批准上市的药物时，他们需要得到批准。测试可能包括这些药物的新剂量或新应用。

当公司开发一种新药时，在向公众销售前必须要得到食品和药物管理局的批准。公司必须通过一系列的步骤和审批才能达到这一点。这取决于也被称之为药品投资商的公司所进行的必要测试、收集数据，并确保病人在服用药物时不会暴露在不必要的风险之下。食品和药物管理局会在每个阶段后审查结果，并确定该药物对公众是否安全。

试验性药物的临床试验阶段是最为重要的。如果食品和药物管理局批准了该试验性新药的申请，这个研究药物将进入临床试验的三个阶段：

第一阶段：用一年左右的时间对约 20～80 名健康志愿者建立药物的安全性和概述。同时强调药物的安全性、代谢和排泄。

第二阶段：在特定条件或疾病中，约 100 到 300 名病人志愿者来评估药物的有效性。这个阶段大约持续 2 年。一组相似的病人可能会接受实际药物与安慰剂（无活性药丸）或其他活性药物的比较，以确定药物是否有效果。并审查其安全性和副作用。

第三阶段：通常，几千名患者在诊所和医院的监测下，谨慎的确定药物有效性和更多的副作用。评估包含不同类型和年龄段的患者。制造商可能会研究不同的剂量和试验药物与其他治疗方法的结合。这个阶段平均大约持续 3 年。

要把一种新药推向市场，进行临床试验可能要历经很多年并花费数亿美元。试验性新药申请表明，投资者愿意进行这项巨大的投资。本身，投资者对于试验性新药申请的反应通常是中立的，因为这仅仅是漫长而艰难的药物审批过程中的第一步。

（詹姆斯·陈是投资百科交易与投资部总监）

Unit 7

Keys to Exercises

Warming-up

1. C；2. A；3. D；4. B

Reading A

Task 1

1. Antibiotics for long have been available in the country's hospitals to prevent post-surgery and other infections. They are also available over the counter at drug stores which people use for self-treatment——for conditions like cough or a running nose.

2. The more antibiotics a person has taken the greater the risk he/she has to be infected by superbugs.

3. Becausethe misuse of antibiotics in the agricultural sector is still widespread. For example, some farm operators feed food animals with antibiotics to prevent infection and boost the growth, which has turned the farms into fertile breeding grounds for drug-resistant pathogens that could contaminate the soil and water and migrate to humans through food.

4. Monitor the antibiotics contamination level and help raise public awareness.

5. "AMR" refers to Anti-microbial Resistance which occurs when bacterial, viruses, fungi, and parasites resist the effects of medications.

Task 2

1. c；2. f；3. a；4. d；5. j；6. i；7. e；8. b；9. g；10. h

Task 3

1. misusing；2. banned；3. infect；4. migration；5. prematurely

Task 4

1. Improper or overuse of antibiotics is proven to be the leading cause of public health problems.

2. Imagine you have bacterial infection and all the antibiotics prescribed by doctors in the hospital cannot cure it.

3. Antibiotics are also available over the counter at drugstores which people use for self-treatment——for conditions like cough or a running nose.

4. These antibiotic-resistant genes can contaminate the soil and water.

5. The environment and education authorities will join the fight by monitoring the antibiotics contamination level and helping raise public awareness.

Listening & Speaking

Task 1

Medication Safety Tips: How to Prevent Adverse Drug Events?

Instructor：Hello, I am your instructor today. Do you know what is an adverse drug event?

Student：Yes, drug event is any harm that occurs from using medications. Sometimes the harm is not preventable such as an allergic reaction, but sometimes the harms results from mistakes are preventable,

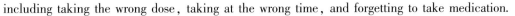

including taking the wrong dose, taking at the wrong time, and forgetting to take medication.

Instructor: Good job. And do you know what kind of people are most at risk for adverse drug events?

Student: The elder people I think.

Instructor: Right, children, the elder adults over 65 years old and anyone who takes multiple medications. Some studies have shown that taking more than four medications puts you at increased risk for an adverse drug event. So, how can we prevent adverse drug events?

Student: When I dispense drugs, I should stick to 'five rights' principle which is the right patient, the right drug, the right dose, the right route and the right time.

Instructor: Additionally, you should teach your patient some medication safety tips. Number one, carry a list of your medications in your wallet. Don't forget to write the allergies and the doctor's phone number and the pharmacist's phone number on the list.

Student: OK.

Instructor: Number two, make detailed instructions in drug use. Moreover, you should clarify the information about drug with the patients.

1. F; 2. T; 3. F; 4. F; 5. T

Task 2

Making an Instruction in Drug Use

Pharmacist: So, I just going to take a few minutes here to show you how to give the medication to your daughter. Did the doctor tell you how much you're giving or how to give the medication?

Patient's mother: No.

Pharmacist: Ok, it's amoxicillin and it's an antibiotic to eradicate the ear infection. First of all, I would recommend storing this in the fridge.

Patient's mother: What will happen if I put them outside of the fridge?

Pharmacist: It will go bad in high temperature.

Pharmacist: And before you give it, you're going to give it a really good shake.

Patient's mother: Shake well?

Pharmacist: Yes, because some of the ingredients settle to the bottom. Drinking the medication without mixing means you will not get desired effects.

Patient's mother: I must write it down on my note book.

Pharmacist: And you're going to give seven mils every 12 hours for a total of 10 days.

Patient's mother: Can I put all seven mils in her mouth at once?

Pharmacist: Please don't do that. Your daughter is still so little and it's her first medication. It can cause aspiration if she takes too many solutions. Do it about two to three installments.

Patient's mother: OK, got it.

Pharmacist: Finally, you should give the medication for the full course of the ten days to make sure the infection clears up even though she's feeling better.

Patient's mother: I don't want my daughter to take so many drugs. They will bring some side effects like liver damage to her.

Pharmacist: The reasons for the full course therapy are that this will stop the infection from returning, as well as reduce the risk of the bacterial becoming resistant to the antibiotics.

Patient's mother: I don't realize it. OK, I will follow the order. Thank you so much.

1. B；2. B；3. D；4. C；5. A

Task 3

In the U. S. , the government's Food and Drug Administration（FDA）must approve any drug before it can be sold. This is true whether it's a <u>prescription</u> or an <u>over-the-counter</u> drug. The FDA evaluates the safety of a drug by looking at side effects：how it's <u>manufactured</u> and results of animal testing and clinical <u>trials.</u> The FDA also <u>monitors</u> a drug's safety after approval. For you，drug safety means buying online from only legitimate pharmacies and taking your medicines correctly.

1. prescription；2. over-the-counter；3. manufactured；4. trials；5. monitors

Reading B

Task 1

1. D；2. D；3. B；4. C；5. B

Task 2

1. 24 小时内服用 4000 毫克的对乙酰氨基酚可导致严重肝损害。

2. 它能暂时缓解关节炎造成的轻微疼痛。

3. 对乙酰氨基酚可导致严重的皮肤反应，如皮肤变红、水疱和皮疹。

4. 如果正在服用血液稀释药物华法林，服用本药前咨询医生或药剂师。

5. 如果出现药物服用过量，立即联系医务人员或中毒控制中心。

Practical Writing

Rosuvastatin Calcium

Generic Name：<u>Rosuvastatin Calcium（Keding）</u>

Trade Name：<u>Rosuvastatin Calcium</u>

Ingredients：<u>molecular formula $(C_{22}H_{27}FN_3O_6S)_2Ca$</u>

Functions and Indications：<u>Hypertriglyceridemia, Primary Dysbetalipoproteinemia, Adult Patients with Homozygous Familial Hypercholesterolemia</u>

Description：<u>Pink, round, biconvex, film-coated tablets</u>

Strength：<u>10mg/tablet ∗7</u>

Administration and Dosage：<u>5mg orally once daily</u>

Adverse Reactions：<u>Headache, asthenia, myalgia, nausea, abdominal pain</u>

Contraindications：You should not take rosuvastatin if you are allergic to it，or if you have

<u>liver disease</u>

<u>kidney disease</u>

<u>if you are pregnant or breast-feeding</u>

Note：See your doctor straight away if you notice any yellowing of <u>your skin or shortness of breath,</u> <u>unexplained cough or general tiredness.</u>

Package：<u>Aluminum /Aluminum plastic foamed package</u>

Storage：<u>Sealed in dry place</u>

Shelf life：<u>36 months</u>

Grammar Tips

Task 1

1. was performed; 2. have been carried out; 3. presents; 4. had gained; 5. had been eating; 6. will have been married; 7. will be falling over; 8. is listening to; 9. were going to visit; 10. admitted

Task 2

1. C; 2. D; 3. A; 4. C; 5. C; 6. C; 7. A; 8. D; 9. A; 10. D

Supplementary Reading

1. T; 2. F; 3. F; 4. T; 5. F

Vocabulary Tips

1. contaminate; 2. Allergic rhinitis; 3. consolidate; 4. Appendicitis; 5. compatriot

Translation for Reference

课文 A

过度使用抗生素对健康的危害

想象一下有一天，你被细菌感染而医生开的所有抗生素都无法治愈。这不是关于"超级细菌"的科幻小说，它实际上正在世界范围内发生。事实证明，抗生素使用不当或过度使用是造成公共卫生问题的主要原因。

中国抗生素滥用的现状

中国使用的抗生素占全球的一半，一半用于人类，其余用于食用动物。长期以来，中国的医院一直在使用抗生素来预防术后感染和其他感染。人们也可以到药店直接买抗生素用于自我治疗，比如治疗咳嗽或者流鼻涕。

根据公共卫生专家的观点，抗生素使用量越多，人类被超级细菌感染的风险就越大。他们敦促政府应协调各部门，一起努力来制止抗生素滥用和应对挑战。

今年在英国出版的《抗微生物药物耐药性评论》（AMR）中提到：预估到 2050 年，中国每年将有 100 万人由于 AMR（包括抗生素抗药性）而早逝。

中国预防 AMR 的协调行动

中国的决策者已经意识到这个迫在眉睫的危机，并决定采取协调一致的行动来预防它。十余个部门（包括原国家卫生和计划生育委员会，原国家食品药品监督管理总局及教育部等）将发布一项有关 AMR 预防和控制的国家级行动计划。

北京大学临床药理研究所肖永红教授说，这项迟来的倡议表明，政府决心正面直击并解决这一问题。

此前，卫生部门在很大程度上采取了抗击 AMR 的措施，其中包括更严格地控制医疗机构对抗生素的使用。例如，2015 年江苏省成为第一个全面禁止对门诊病人使用静脉注射抗生素的省份。江苏省卫生部门表示，随着公众对于过度使用抗生素的认识程度的提高，这个禁令正在奏效。浙江、江西和安徽等其他省份也可能很快效仿江苏这一措施。但这还远远不够抗击 AMR。

许多中国专家甚至在英国有关 AMR 的报告中指出，中国农业领域滥用抗生素的现象仍然很普遍。

为防止食用动物感染疾病并促进它们的生长（大部分食用动物都饲养在满是粪便、拥挤不堪的农场中），农场主定期给它们喂服抗生素。这使农场变成了抗药性病原体的肥沃繁殖地，而这些病原体也能威胁人类。

还记得 2013 年的中美联合研究吗？研究发现"中国养猪场中存在大量多样的耐药基因"，这些基因可能污染土壤和水，并通过食物迁移到人类。因此，如果农业部门不积极采取遏制给食用动物喂食抗生素的措施，就无法赢得抗微生物药物耐药性的斗争。

其他的利益相关部门也必须参与这场斗争，如环境和教育部门可通过监测抗生素污染水平和提高公众意识抗击 AMR。

全球抗击 AMR 的战争需要中国

中国抗击 AMR 还有一条很长的路要走，预期的政府行动计划是针对 AMR 全面开战的良好开端，这也将有助于中国履行其在公共卫生领域的国际责任。中国必须成为全球抗微生物药物耐药性斗争的一部分。没有中国，就不可能赢得全球性抗击 AMR 的战争。

课文 B

泰诺的药品说明书

强力泰诺——对乙酰氨基酚片，薄膜片

纳瓦霍制造有限公司

药名

通用名：对乙酰氨基酚

商品名：泰诺

有效成分（每囊片）

对乙酰氨基酚 500 毫克

用药目的

缓解疼痛/退热

适应证

➢ 暂时缓解由于以下原因引起的轻微疼痛：

·普通感冒　　　　·头痛　　　　·腰痛

·关节炎的轻微疼痛　·牙痛　　　　·肌肉酸痛

·月经前和月经期的疼痛

➢ 暂时退热

警告

肝损害：本产品含有对乙酰氨基酚。如果按照以下方式服用，可导致严重肝损害：

· 24 小时内服用 4000 毫克的对乙酰氨基酚

· 同时服用其他含有对乙酰氨基酚的药物

· 使用本品时，同时每天服用 3 种或以上的酒精饮料

过敏反应：对乙酰氨基酚可导致严重的皮肤反应。症状可包括：

·皮肤变红 · 水疱· 皮疹

如果出现皮肤反应，立即停止用药并联系医务人员

有以下情况，请勿使用：

· 正在服用还有对乙酰氨基酚的其他药物（处方药或非处方药）。如果不确定药物是否含有对乙酰氨基酚，咨询医生或药剂师。

· 如果您对对乙酰氨基酚或本产品中的任何非活性成分过敏

如果患有肝病，使用前请咨询医生。

如果正在服用血液稀释药物华法林，使用前咨询医生或药剂师。

有以下情况，停止用药并咨询医生：

· 疼痛加重或持续 10 天以上

· 发热加重或持续 3 天以上

· 出现新的症状

· 出现发红或肿胀

以上症状可能表明情况很严重。

如果怀孕或哺乳，使用前咨询医生。

请将本药品放在儿童不能接触的地方。

过量警告：如果出现药物服用过量，立即联系医务人员或中毒控制中心。（电话：1 – 800 – 222 – 1222）即使没有发现任何症状和体征，快速的医疗护理不仅对于儿童非常重要，对于成年人也非常重要。

用药指导

	· 不要超过规定剂量（请看过量警告）
成人和 12 岁及以上儿童	· 每 6 小时服用 2 片药（伴随有症状时） · 除非有医生要求，否则 24 小时内不要超过 6 片药 · 除非有医生要求，用药不能超过 10 天
12 岁以下儿童	· 咨询医生

其他信息

· 保存温度为 20 ~ 25°C（68 ~ 77°F）

· 批号和有效期见盒子底部

· 如果包装破损请勿使用

非活性成分

巴西棕榈蜡＊，玉米淀粉，食用红色编号 40 铝色淀，羟丙甲纤维素，硬脂酸镁，聚乙二醇＊，粉状纤维素，预胶化淀粉，丙二醇，虫胶，羟乙酸淀粉钠，二氧化钛。

＊包含一种或多种这些成分

问题或意见？

致电 1 – 877 – 895 – 3665（免费电话）或 215 – 273 – 8755（对方收费）

补充阅读

非处方药物的滥用，你需要了解它的一切

当我们想到药物滥用和药物成瘾时，我们经常想到非法的毒品。但是，2018 年 5 月美国食品和药物管理局博客中，局长 Scott Gottlieb 对越来越多的人滥用和过度使用非处方药（OTC）发出警告。非处方药是无需处方即可获得的药物，在药店和超市均有出售。

如果按照推荐剂量和推荐用药周期使用，这些药物是安全的。但是，与非法药物和处方药一样，非处方药也可能被滥用。OTC 药物滥用的最常见形式包括服用剂量高于推荐剂量，服用时间长于推荐用药时间，以及将它们与其他药物混合以制成新产品。尽管它们的效力（按用药指南服用）不如非法药物强，但 OTC 药物仍具有成瘾的风险。

哪些是最常见滥用的 OTC 药物?

· 止咳药和感冒药（右美沙芬）

· 止痛药（对乙酰氨基酚和布洛芬）

· 鼻血管收缩药（伪麻黄碱）

· 晕车药（苯海拉明）

· 止泻药（洛哌丁胺）

· 减肥药（麻黄碱）

· 非处方助眠剂/安眠药（苯海拉明）

滥用非处方药有多危险?

据美国国家药物滥用研究所/美国国立卫生研究院称,许多经常滥用的非处方药,包括咳嗽药、止泻药、晕车药和减肥药,可能会导致严重甚至危及生命的症状。

不幸的是,由于这些药物可以通过非处方药获得,因此人们常常对它们有一种错误的安全感。

人们滥用非处方药物可出于娱乐目的,也可因为疏忽大意,比如不认真遵循用药指南。但是他们这样做的风险比想象的要大。

咳嗽药物滥用

滥用止咳药会导致头晕、恶心、呕吐、呼吸和视力问题,癫痫发作和焦虑/惊恐症状。当同时服用含有右美沙芬的止咳药和非处方止痛药对乙酰氨基酚时,可能会发生肝损害。

非处方止痛药滥用

非处方止痛药,例如对乙酰氨基酚,通常用于缓解疼痛和退热。对乙酰氨基酚的滥用通常是由于尝试不使用阿片类药物治疗慢性疼痛而引起的。

滥用 OTC 止痛药的危险是过量服用会严重损害肝脏。

鼻血管收缩药（伪麻黄碱）滥用

过量服用鼻血管收缩药会导致血压升高,心跳加快至危险水平,并导致心律不齐,癫痫发作或幻觉。

非处方助眠剂/安眠药

根据食品和药物管理局的药物标签,苯海拉明可引起便秘、意识障碍、眩晕和第二天的嗜睡。根据《消费者报告》的评论,另一个令人担忧的问题是该药物的"宿醉效应"——即服用该药物后的第二天,平衡、协调和驾驶能力受损,这可能会增加跌倒和发生事故的风险。

滥用非处方药是危险的行为

乍一看,使用非处方药似乎是安全无忧的,但使用者应慎重用药。在这里,古希腊人的警示语"万事有度"是非常合适的。非处方药也是药物,而且其有效成分具有强大的效力。滥用或误用这些产品（例如过量服用）可能与使用非法药物一样有害和危险。

Unit 8

Keys to Exercises

Warming-up

1. B; 2. D; 3. A; 4. C

Reading A

Task 1

1. In 2016, China became the world's second largest pharmaceutical market and the total sales reached almost CYN 28 billion.

2. Because the average revenue and the middle class in China are growing.

3. It aims to enable patients to choose between hospitals and retail pharmacies for prescription drug purchases.

4. E-commerce is also creating opportunity and way for new pharmaceutical brands to sell their products in China. The online pharmacy can promote new brands and new products to customers, creating their needs.

5. Because of the very complex distribution chain in China, drug prices used to be very high. Selling on online platforms allows customers to get fairer prices.

Task 2

1. g; 2. d; 3. c; 4. a; 5. f; 6. b; 7. h; 8. i; 9. j; 10. e

Task 3

1. evolve; 2. necessity; 3. Distribution; 4. giants; 5. competitor

Task 4

1. According to China Food and Drug Administration (CFDA), in 2017, 659 online pharmacies obtained the permission.

2. Hospitals were the main place to get drugs and they counted on drug sales for revenue.

3. It aims to enable patients to choose between hospitals and retail pharmacies for prescription drug purchases.

4. E-commerce is also creating opportunity and way for new pharmaceutical brands to sell their products in China.

5. Tmall and Jingdong are the most reliable platforms for a major part of Chinese consumers.

Listening & Speaking

Task 1

I'd Like to Introduce My Colleague

Zhang: Excuse me, but aren't you Mr. David Smith, the sales manager from ABC Pharmaceutical Company?

Smith: Yes, I am. And you are···

Zhang: I'm Zhang Yang from Sinopharm. We met at 2019 London International Health Expo.

Smith: Ah, yes. I remember now.

Zhang: It's nice to see you again, Mr. Smith.

Smith: Nice to see you again, too.

Zhang: Mr. Smith, I'd like to introduce my colleague, Mr. Wang Jun, the marketing manager of our company.

Smith：How do you do, Mr. Wang? It's my pleasure to meet you.

Wang：How do you do, Mr. Smith? The pleasure is mine.

Smith：Here's my business card.

Wang：Thanks. And here's mine.

1. F；2. F；3. T；4. F；5. T

Task 2

What's on the Cards for Tomorrow's General Meeting?

Robert：Mike, what's on the cards for tomorrow's general meeting?

Mike：I think one of our sales representatives is going to give us a rundown on our most recent sales figures.

Robert：Is everyone going to be there?

Mike：As far as I know everyone will be there.

Robert：I hope so, this will be important for company's near-term future.

Mike：Robert, maybe we should double check to make sure everyone is aware of the importance of this meeting.

Robert：Leave that to my secretary. I'll get her onto it.

Mike：Will I need to organize someone from the marketing department to give us their viewpoint on the sales results?

Robert：Yes, actually that's quite a good idea considering that it was their marketing campaign that ultimately resulted in the products success or failure.

Mike：OK, I'll organize that for tomorrow's meeting then. I hope they will be able to prepare something on such a short notice.

1. B；2. C；3. B；4. A；5. D

Task 3

"Pharmacoeconomics" is a new word; but economic interest in drug and other treatments of <u>health</u> problems is much older. <u>Decisions</u> about what treatments should be appropriate within a health care system have always been influenced by the resources <u>available</u> to pay for them. Pharmacoeconomics can be <u>defined</u> as the branch of economics that uses cost-benefit, cost-effectiveness, cost-minimization, cost-of-illness and cost-utility analyses to compare pharmaceutical <u>products</u> and treatment strategies.

1. health；2. Decisions；3. available；4. defined；5. products

Reading B

Task 1

1. D；2. C；3. B；4. D；5. A

Task 2

1. 营销策略帮助企业实现经营目标，而营销组合（4Ps）是定义营销策略的常用框架。

2. 除此之外，第三类产品包括作物科学，主要研究高价值种子，最佳病虫害防治方案，并对客户的农用方法给予指导服务。

3. 因此，能按照既定的全球标准遵循安全和环境安全守则，此外也能降低成本，使运输体系流畅。

4. 环境、社会和治理标准决定是否与现有供应商继续合作。

5. 它以足球俱乐部而闻名，但也参与排球、拳击、篮球和田径等其他各种运动。

Practical Writing

Report on Effective Team Leadership

The aim of this report is to summarize the recent Team Leadership Workshop and recommend appropriate action.

It was discovered that the team leaders had different understandings of their roles based on the assessment during the workshop. Having identified the different possible approaches to each key task, the company was able to select which was most appropriate in terms of skills and behavior required.

To conclude, we can see that the company needs to ensure that its team leaders are capable of performing key tasks compatible with company expectations. Therefore, we strongly recommend the company should immediately set up an assessment center where team leaders can be evaluated to ensure that they have the characteristics for effective team leadership.

Barrie Watson

Grammar Tips

Task 1

1. （should） take；2. （should） be appointed；3. （should） know；4. would have been understood；5. had been；6. went / should go；7. should happen / were to happen / happened；8. would have had to leave；9. would have worked；10. （should） be raised

Task 2

1. B；2. D；3. C；4. C；5. C；6. B；7. C；8. A；9. C；10. D

Supplementary Reading

1. F；2. T；3. F；4. F；5. T

Vocabulary Tips

1. dermatitis；2. arthroncus；3. hemorrhage；4. hypodermic；5. Hemodiagnosis

Translation for Reference

课文 A

中国网上药店，前景光明的售药方式

医药行业是中国的主要产业之一。中国于 2005 年开始网上药店经营。2008 年，只有 10 家网

上药店获准销售药品。根据原国家食品药品监督管理总局（CDFA）的数据，2017 年，659 家网上药店获得了经营许可。不仅药店数量激增，销量也在蓬勃发展。中康咨询的研究数据表明，2016 年 B2C 电子药房的销售额同比增长了 93%，达到近 280 亿元。2016 年，中国成为世界第二大医药市场。

中国医药市场

随着中国平均收入和中产阶级的增长，对医疗保健产品和服务的需求越来越大。老一辈人想为孩子存钱，所以只在自己身上花很少的钱。新一代人更关心自己，也更关心家人。对他们来说，在身体或医疗保健上花钱是必要的，也是常态。

全国连锁药店覆盖了医药市场。医院是获取药品的主要场所，其依靠药品销售获得收入。政府的新规定允许中国电商巨头涉足医药领域，将处方药销售从医院转向零售。其目的是使患者在购买处方药时可在医院和零售药店之间选择。

必须赶上电子药房的发展

中国电子商务市场的快速增长与该领域的许多新规定及不同的新竞争者进入该领域有关。这个市场的竞争日益激烈，使得折扣网上药店在其中占据重要一席。由于市场正处于快速发展阶段，前景非常乐观。每年平均增长 30% 左右。

电子商务也为新的医药品牌在中国销售产品创造了机会和途径。网上药店可以向顾客推广新品牌、新产品，创造顾客的需求。网上折扣多，对用户会更有吸引力，用户也能花时间去发现它们。对于大部分中国消费者来说，天猫和京东是最为可靠的平台。

医药行业的未来在网上

现实是一个可靠的电子商务平台可以让消费者放心购买他们的药品。随着电子商务的发展，中国人改变了购买药品的习惯。电子商务变得越来越重要有很多原因：

·由于中国的分销链非常复杂，过去药品价格很高。在网络平台销售可以让消费者获得更公道的价格。通过这种方式，信息也更加透明。

·80% 的中国年轻人已经在网上研究过相关医疗信息。他们在网上参与讨论，并在网上寻求药物的建议或推荐。他们可获得不同建议并进行比较。

·由于处于强度高、压力大的工作环境，中国人寻求如何节约时间并提高效率。如今快递服务在中国非常发达。因此，网上购物和去药店一样方便（甚至更方便）。客户不受营业时间限制。

课文 B

拜耳营销组合（4Ps）策略

拜耳的营销组合策略分析品牌或公司，包括 4P（产品、价格、地点、促销），并解释拜耳的营销策略。截至 2020 年，有多种营销策略，如产品/服务创新、营销投资、客户体验等，这些策略都有助于品牌的发展。

营销策略帮助企业实现经营目标，而营销组合（4Ps）是定义营销策略的常用框架。以下是 4Ps 策略，详细阐述了拜耳使用的产品、定价、分销和广告策略。

拜耳产品策略

拜耳为其客户提供种类繁多的产品。有一些主要品牌构成拜耳营销产品组合策略的一部分。这些产品有助于找到给我们带来巨大挑战的解决方案。它们主要分为四类。药品类包括妇女保健、心脏病、肿瘤学和血液学的处方药。拜耳最畅销的产品包括拜科奇、倍泰龙、抑肽酶和齐普罗。另一个类别是健康消费品。这些产品主要包括皮肤病、过敏性疾病、咳嗽感冒、足部护理和防晒护理的非处方产品。除此之外,第三类产品包括作物科学,主要研究高价值种子,最佳病虫害防治方案,并对客户的农用方法给予指导服务。动物保健类包括为农场动物和伴生动物提供产品。

拜耳价格/定价策略

定价在医药行业中占有重要地位。拜耳一直专注于高质量产品。为了保持高质量,价格成为重要因素。拜耳一直遵循基于竞争的营销组合定价策略。其大多数产品的价格都与竞争对手产品价格相似。但是,区别因素是他们在质量上从未妥协。拜耳有自己的采购网点。因此,能按照既定的全球标准遵循安全和环境安全守则,此外也能降低成本,使运输体系流畅。

拜耳渠道与分销策略

渠道管理对拜耳而言非常重要。这就保证其能在正确的时间和地点提供所需商品和服务。这有助于在分销渠道中物料的持续平稳供应。在为产品选择供应商时,拜耳尤为苛刻。其制定了自己独有的行为准则,即拜耳供应商行为准则。环境、社会和治理标准决定是否与现有供应商继续合作。目前,这些供应商将产品销往多个合格零售商,最终经由这些零售商到达客户手中。

拜耳宣传与广告策略

拜耳创立了名为拜耳04勒沃库森的体育俱乐部。它以足球俱乐部而闻名,但也参与排球、拳击、篮球和田径等其他各种运动。勒沃库森是德国最大的体育俱乐部之一。拜耳还赞助了多尔马根、伍珀塔尔等俱乐部。拜耳在脸书、推特、油管、领英和照片墙等各种社交媒体平台都有业务。其还推出了电子贺卡,可以通过拜耳世界免费发送给你的亲人。这也涵盖了拜耳营销组合。

补充阅读

医药行业销售与营销

背景

医药行业的销售与营销是指为临床方面及获得市场份额而推广药品的商业活动。某些方面侧重于分析特定市场需求的能力,其他方面则偏向开发特定疗法和产品交流。

该领域的从业者遵循受全行业支持的指导方针和规则。美国医药研究制药协会(PhRMA)在几年前为销售和营销人员制定了一套行为守则。以下信息可大致了解美国医药研究制药协会行为守则所涉及的范围:

1. 禁止企业销售代表向医护人员提供餐饮服务,但允许其在进行资料展示时,在医护人员办公室偶尔提供膳食。

2. 包括新的规定,要求企业确保其代表在适用法律、法规、行业实践守则和道德规范方面得到充分培训。

3. 规定每家企业都要声明愿意遵守该守则,首席执行官和监察官员每年都要证明有适当的流程可供遵守。

4. 包括关于继续医学教育独立性的更详细标准。

5. 为与医护人员的谈话和咨询提供额外的指导和约束。

美国医药研究制药协会行为守则——2009修订指南

除了传统的电话销售外,还出现了新的通讯工具。社交媒体技术正在改变医药营销过程。与多媒体合作的机会开启了新的营销策略和销售计划。

最吸引人之处

27%的受访从业者提到，这些角色中最吸引人的一个方面是他们对病人的影响。对许多人来说，这是这个职业的间接优势。同样的百分比还表明，一个吸引人之处是与医护人员（药剂师、医生、护士或其他人）一起工作合作。

一名受访者表示"喜欢与整个医疗市场的临床医生互动"。另一名受访者很享受"与药剂师和护士一起工作以提高病人安全感并节约成本"。

13%的人认为工作环境是最吸引人的方面之一。许多公司的办公室都很现代化，有供员工使用的便利设施。其中一位员工评论"工作环境非常好"。

最不吸引人之处

有18%的从业者认为官僚和政治是最不吸引人的方面。这些从业者对自己的工作非常满意，但一位受访者认为"行政工作和大公司政治"是这份工作最不吸引人之处。9%的受访者提到了文书工作和差旅。一名受访者表示不喜欢"差旅和远离临床实践"。

Unit 9

Keys to Exercises

Warming-up

1. D; 2. C; 3. B; 4. A

Reading A

Task 1

1. In 1581, the first Spanish Pharmacopoeias appeared in Europe.

2. The breakthrough progress in the 19th century life sciences, especially in chemistry, physiology and pharmacology facilitated the development of modern medicines regulation.

3. Registration of drugs is the most important element of medication regulation.

4. Effective medicines regulation demands the application of sound medical, scientific and technical knowledge and skills, and operates within a legal framework.

5. All medicines must meet three criteria: be of good quality, safe and effective.

Task 2

1. e; 2. a; 3. d; 4. h; 5. j; 6. i; 7. c; 8. b; 9. f; 10. g

Task 3

1. pharmacopoeia; 2. Foundation; 3. flourishing; 4. distribution; 5. implement

Task 4

1. All drugs that are marketed, distributed and used in the country should be registered by the national competent regulatory authority.

2. Drug regulation should include the scientific evaluation of products before registration, to ensure that all marketed pharmaceutical products meet the criteria of safety, efficacy and quality.

3. Consumers are not in a position to weigh potential benefits against risks as no medicine is completely safe.

4. In broad terms the mission of NRAs is to protect and promote public health.

5. The judgments about medicines quality, safety and efficacy should be based on solid science.

Listening & Speaking

Task 1

Food Poisoning

Doctor: What's wrong with you?

Bob: I have a bad stomachache.

Doctor: Where does the pain start?

Bob: I have pain in the right lower stomach and upper abdomen.

Doctor: Did it spread to other parts of the body or not?

Bob: No, it does not spread to other parts.

Doctor: Does the pain come and go or is it constant?

Bob: It is constant, but sharpens at times, like a needle prick.

Doctor: Have you got diarrhea or vomit?

Bob: Yes, I have been having diarrhea and keep vomiting.

Doctor: Did you eat something strange?

Bob: Nothing special, oh··· I had spaghetti with clam sauce for breakfast.

Doctor: Do you think that maybe you are getting the food poisoning?

Bob: It could be bad food, but I didn't feel so bad for the past few hours.

Doctor: Most food borne illness symptoms don't present right away. It often takes 24 to 48 hours after eating the contaminated food. I need to give you a thorough examination···

1. T; 2. F; 3. F; 4. T; 5. F

Task 2

What FDA Is Doing to Protect Consumers?

Reporter: What contaminants are we talking about?

Conrad Choiniere: A reality about our food supply is that metals, such as arsenic, lead, cadmium, mercury and others are present in certain foods.

Reporter: Would you say more about how they get into our food supply?

Conrad Choiniere: These elements occur naturally and as environmental pollutants in air, water and soil and they enter the food supply when plants take them up as they grow.

Reporter: Can you describe the work the group is doing?

Conrad Choiniere: Part of the work involves studying the large amount of data FDA has collected over the years. We have been collecting data on contaminants and nutrients in foods for decades as part of our Total Diet Study.

Reporter：What actions will follow all this data collecting and analyses?

Conrad Choiniere：FDA is working to protect consumers of all ages from these metals when present in foods.

Reporter：We've talked about kids, but what about the elderly and other populations? Is the workgroup looking out for them too?

Conrad Choiniere：Certainly, children are one of our most vulnerable populations, but we are concerned about the health of all populations, including older consumers and people who may have chronic health conditions.

Repoter：What drives you to do this work?

Conrad Choiniere：I eat food, and I have children too. Protecting kids and vulnerable populations is important to me and I'm fortunate to work with very dedicated people who feel the same way and who do their best to protect people and the food we eat.

1. B；2. A；3. B；4. D；5. C

Task 3

Keeping the family safe is a priority in any household. Being smart about how we shop for food can do a lot to help prevent exposure to the two most common food borne agents：viruses and bacteria . When it comes to food borne illness, most of us think of under-cooked meat and eggs. But the raw fruits and vegetables can pose a risk, so can lunch, meat and deli-type salads. There are a few things you can do while at the grocery store：check the sell-by dates, use plastic bags for raw meat and poultry and keep them separated from the other groceries in your cart, and only buy pasteurized dairy products and juice.

1. safe；2. viruses；3. bacteria；4. risk；5. dairy

Reading B

Task 1

1. C；2. D；3. A；4. D；5. B

Task 2

1. 国家药品监督管理局是中国政府负责药品、医疗器械和化妆品监管的行政机构。

2. 国家药品监督管理局负责药品（含中药、民族药，下同）、医疗器械和化妆品安全监督管理。

3. 国家药品监督管理局负责药品、医疗器械和化妆品标准管理。

4. 国家药品监督管理局组织开展药品不良反应、医疗器械不良事件和化妆品不良反应的监测、评价和处置工作。

5. 国家药品监督管理局负责制定检查制度，依法查处药品、医疗器械和化妆品注册环节的违法行为，依职责组织指导查处生产环节的违法行为。

Practical Writing

Business Letters

RED EAST INTERNATIONAL Ltd.

REGISTERED ADDRESS: 18 SOUTH STREET, JING AN DISTRICT SHANGHAI, 200040

PHONE: 86-021-62888888   FAX: 86-021-62888866   WEBSITE: www. redeast. com

March 20, 2020

Sales Manager

Westin Corporation

20 West Street, Brooklyn

New York, 10268

U. S. A

Dear R. James,

Thank you for your letter of March 15. It's our pleasure to establish business relations with your company.

We are delighted to send you the information you need. The attached catalogue will give you full details and prices of the goods we can supply, and you will find the quality and price are competitive. We await your information with interest.

Yours truly,

RED EAST INTERNATIONAL Ltd.

(Signature)

Zhang Lin

Marketing Manager

Grammar Tips

Task 1

1. shows; 2. are; 3. is; 4. look; 5. is; 6. wants; 7. was; 8. is; 9. has; 10. is

Task 2

1. A; 2. B; 3. C; 4. A; 5. C; 6. B; 7. D; 8. C; 9. B; 10. A

Supplementary Reading

1. F; 2. T; 3. T; 4. F; 5. T

Vocabulary Tips

1. macrocosm; 2. discriminate; 3. dispassionate; 4. dissect; 5. cosmetic

Translation for Reference

课文 A

药品监管

药品监管历史

药物可能和人类一样古老，如何保证其质量的观念随着时间的推移而逐渐演变。直到 1540 年，英格兰的药品生产才受到《药剂师货品、药品和物品法》的监管。这可以看作是药品检查的开始。作为药物质量标准的官方书籍，药典的历史可以追溯到西西里岛弗雷德里克二世（1240 年）颁布的萨莱诺医学法令之一。我们今天所知道的第一个药典是从 16 世纪开始出现在欧洲的。例如，第一部西班牙药典是在 1581 年发行的。

现代药品监管是在 19 世纪生命科学特别是化学、生理学和药理学取得突破性进展后开始的，为现代药物研发奠定了坚实的基础，并在第二次世界大战后开始蓬勃发展。

药品注册

药品注册，又称产品许可或销售许可，是药品监管的重要组成部分。凡在国内销售、分销和使用的药品，必须经国家药品监管部门注册。

药品监管应包括注册前对产品进行科学评估，以确保所有上市的药品都安全、有效，并符合质量标准。这些标准适用于所有药物，包括生物制品（含疫苗、血液制品、单克隆抗体、细胞和组织疗法）和草药。

为什么要进行药品监管?

药物不是普通消费者的产品。在大多数情况下，由于没有一种药物是完全安全的，消费者无法决定何时使用药物、使用哪些药物、如何使用药物，以及权衡潜在的益处和风险。在做这些决定时，需要处方师或药剂师的专业建议。

因此，各国政府需要建立强有力的国家监管部门（NRAs），以确保药品的生产、贸易和使用得到有效监管。从广义上讲，国家监管部门的任务是保护和促进公众健康。

如何确保药品监管有效?

药品监管要求应用健全的医疗、科学及技术的知识与技能，并在法律框架内运作。监管职能涉及与各种利益攸关方（例如制造商、贸易商、消费者、卫生专业人员、研究人员和政府）的相互作用，这些利益攸关方的经济、社会和政治动机可能不同，这使得监管的实施在政治上和技术上都具有挑战性。所有药物必须符合三个标准：质量好、安全和有效。对药品质量、安全性和疗效的判断应以科学为基础。

课文 B

国家药品监督管理局

什么是 NMPA?

国家药品监督管理局（NMPA），是中国政府负责药品、医疗器械和化妆品监管的行政机构。

国家药品监督管理局的职责是什么？

国家药品监督管理局是国家市场监督管理总局下属的副部级行政管理机构。具体来说，国家药品监督管理局负责以下 10 项职能，以监管中国内地市场的药品、医疗器械和化妆品：

（一）负责药品（含中药、民族药，下同）、医疗器械和化妆品安全监督管理。拟订监督管理政策规划，组织起草法律法规草案，拟订部门规章，并监督实施。研究拟订鼓励药品、医疗器械和化妆品新技术新产品的管理与服务政策。

（二）负责药品、医疗器械和化妆品标准管理。组织制定、公布国家药典等药品、医疗器械标准，组织拟订化妆品标准，组织制定分类管理制度，并监督实施。参与制定国家基本药物目录，配合实施国家基本药物制度。

（三）负责药品、医疗器械和化妆品注册管理。制定注册管理制度，严格上市审评审批，完善审评审批服务便利化措施，并组织实施。

（四）负责药品、医疗器械和化妆品质量管理。制定研制质量管理规范并监督实施。制定生产质量管理规范并依职责监督实施。制定经营、使用质量管理规范并指导实施。

（五）负责药品、医疗器械和化妆品上市后风险管理。组织开展药品不良反应、医疗器械不良事件和化妆品不良反应的监测、评价和处置工作。依法承担药品、医疗器械和化妆品安全应急管理工作。

（六）负责执业药师资格准入管理。制定执业药师资格准入制度，指导监督执业药师注册工作。

（七）负责组织指导药品、医疗器械和化妆品监督检查。制定检查制度，依法查处药品、医疗器械和化妆品注册环节的违法行为，依职责组织指导查处生产环节的违法行为。

（八）负责药品、医疗器械和化妆品监督管理领域对外交流与合作，参与相关国际监管规则和标准的制定。

（九）负责指导省、自治区、直辖市药品监督管理部门工作。

（十）完成党中央、国务院交办的其他任务。

补充阅读

中国的社会医疗保险和全民医疗

中国的社会医疗保险是什么样的？

为了到 2020 年实现全民健康覆盖，中国实施了完善医疗保险的全面改革。中国有三种基本医疗保险制度：城镇职工基本医疗保险、城镇居民基本医疗保险和新型农村合作医疗。

在我国，城镇职工基本医疗保险是一种强制性保险，医保费用由用人单位和职工共同承担。尽管各地市的比例可能有所不同，一般是用人单位缴纳工资基数的 6%，个人缴纳工资基数的 2%。灵活就业人员也可以享受医保，但必须全额缴纳。

对于非企业居民，医疗保险由个人和政府支付。对于无业居民和社会救助对象，由国家提供保险补贴。

新型农村合作医疗制度是由中央政府提出的，旨在资助那些因患重病或受伤而面临高额医疗费用的农民。它是一个由政府、集体和个人组成的多渠道筹资体系。

社会医疗保险具体包括什么？

基本医疗保险一般包括：住院治疗、初级保健和专业保健、处方药、精神卫生保健、物理治疗、急救护理和中药。

共同支付、自付和报销比例

不同的保险计划、地区、医院类型（社区、二级或三级），以及其他因素会导致免赔额、自付额和报销封顶线各不相同。因此，包括处方药在内的住院护理和门诊护理的报销均有不同：

门诊诊查费：虽然主任医生诊查费的自付比例较高，但普通门诊诊查费通常较低（5～10元）。处方药报销比例不同：2018年，北京不同医院的报销比例是在药品费用的50%～80%之间。医疗费的报销：住院报销比例远高于门诊服务。

社会医疗保险项目只为病人报销具一定上限的费用，若超过这个上限，居民必须支付所有的自付费用。对于自费支出，没有年度上限。门诊报销上限明显低于住院报销。例如，2018年，北京拥有城镇居民基本医疗保险的居民门诊报销封顶线为3000元。相比之下，住院治疗的报销上限为20万元人民币。报销前必须先扣除年度免赔额，门诊和住院报销的年度免赔额或有不同。

预防服务医疗，如癌症筛查和流感疫苗接种，属于独立的公共卫生项目。医保全面覆盖了儿童与老人的预防医疗费用，但其他居民必须全额自付其预防医疗费用。

人们可以享受异地医疗服务（甚至跨省），但这些服务的自费比例较高。

安全网

对于那些无力缴纳社会医疗保险个人保费或无法支付自付费用的个人，则由地方政府和社会救助机构所资助的医疗财政援助计划为城乡居民提供医疗安全保障。

如何提供医疗保健？

初级保健主要由以下机构提供：

农村诊所的医生和社区卫生工作者。

乡镇和城市社区医院的全科医生或家庭医生。

二、三级医院的医务人员（医生和护士）。

Unit 10

Keys to Exercises

Warming-up

1. B；2. C；3. D；4. A

Reading A

Task 1

1. In healthcare, digital transformation disrupts business models, services, regulations, and skills supply and demand.

2. The Chinese government's overarching idea is to move from "disease-centered" care to "big health".

3. Three digital databases will incorporate health information, health profiles and medical records.

4. Because the Chinese people are already using connected-care technology to track their own health.

5. Wider adoption of smart, connected technologies will boost affordability and access.

Task 2

1. g; 2. d; 3. i; 4. a; 5. j; 6. c; 7. b; 8. h; 9. f; 10. e

Task 3

1. transformation; 2. emphasize; 3. deteriorate; 4. acceleration; 5. denial

Task 4

1. The so-called Fourth Industrial Revolution is in full swing, bringing with it both disruption and opportunity.

2. The Chinese people and healthcare professionals alike recognize the importance of prevention in healthcare.

3. The government has little to do to convince the general public about the benefits of health-related technology.

4. They are already using connected-care technology to track their own health.

5. Wider adoption of smart, connected technologies will continue to boost affordability and access.

Listening & Speaking

Task 1

What are the symptoms of COVID-19?

Daniela: Hi, Elizabeth. COVID-19 has affected every continent in the world. What are the symptoms of patients affected by the disease?

Elizabeth: There can be a range of symptoms from mild to severe. Some people may not develop symptoms.

Daniela: What are the common symptoms?

Elizabeth: Common symptoms include fever, fatigue and respiratory symptoms, such as cough, sore throat and shortness of breath.

Daniela: What about some other symptoms?

Elizabeth: Some people also reported the loss of their sense of taste or smell. And some may develop a skin rash.

Daniela: What are the symptoms of severe patients?

Elizabeth: In severe cases, there could be pneumonia, organ failure, and sometimes death.

1. T; 2. F; 3. T; 4. F; 5. T

Task 2

How to Prevent Transmission of COVID-19?

Daniela：Elizabeth, is there any method for us to prevent COVID-19 from spreading?

Elizabeth：Yes. There are a number of effective ways to prevent the spread of the disease.

Daniela：What can we do to prevent transmission?

Elizabeth：Wear a mask when you are with someone else. Wash your hands regularly with soap and running water or an alcohol-based hand rub.

Daniela：But I have to go out sometimes. What should I do when I am out?

Elizabeth：Keep at least 1 meter distance from people. Cover your mouth and nose when coughing or sneezing with a flexed elbow or tissue. And throw the tissue in a closed bin immediately after use.

Daniela：What if I don't feel well?

Elizabeth：It's important to stay home if you are feeling unwell and to call a hotline. If you have a fever, cough or difficulty breathing, seek medical care early and share your travel history or contact with someone unwell with your healthcare provider.

1. C；2. B；3. C；4. C；5. D

Task 3

If an antibody test finds antibodies in the blood, it likely means the person has been <u>previously</u> infected with the virus. Antibody tests do not show if you have a <u>current</u> infection and should not be used to diagnose a current infection from COVID-19.

The results from antibody tests can help us better understand questions about <u>exposure</u> to COVID-19 by helping identify：who has been infected and has developed antibodies；if antibodies may provide protection from future infection；who may still be at risk；or who may be <u>eligible</u> to donate a part of their blood called convalescent plasma, which may serve as a possible <u>treatment</u> for those who are seriously ill from COVID-19.

1. previously；2. current；3. exposure；4. eligible；5. treatment

Reading B

Task 1

1. D；2. A；3. B；4. D；5. C

Task 2

1. 制药领域自动化和机器人技术的整合大大改善了药品分发的安全性、库存管理和标签功能。

2. 自动化超越了最专注和专业的药剂师的专业技能和知识。

3. 药剂师可以通过整合自动化呼叫程序来显著降低这类风险，这些程序只为患者提供指令性信息。

4. 配药和包装机器人根据要求执行不同的任务。

5. 药房自动化已经改变了传统社区药房以往的工作方式。

Practical Writing

The Situation of General Practitioner Education after Graduation in Chongqing from 2015 to 2018

[Abstract] Objective Through an in-depth analysis of the situation of GP education after graduation in Chongqing from 2015 to 2018, this paper tries to find out the existing problems and put forward some suggestions. Methods The age, education background, identity, certification status and job position of GPs and assistant GPs participating in training from 2015 to 2018 in 55 GP training bases in Chongqing were collected. And the training scale and situation were analyzed. Results From 2015 to 2018, the general practitioner standardized training, and the education background of the participants was mainly undergraduate, accounting for 92.53% of the total number. In 2018, the number of undergraduates was 95.24%, an increase of 5.82% compared with 89.42% in 2015. The participants were mainly fresh graduates and unit personnel, accounting for 60%-70% of the total number of fresh students, and mainly rural order oriented training students, accounting for about 80%. In 2016-2018, the training of assistant general practitioners was mainly based on junior college education, accounting for 98.99% of the total number; among the participants, the fresh graduates accounted for 58.67% of the total number. Conclusion At present, the training of assistant GPs starts late and the scale is insufficient. In the next step, we should continue to carry out training for rural order-oriented students (undergraduates) of clinical medicine and local specialized medical students freely. At the same time, specialized training for medical students should be started as soon as possible, and the training scale of assistant GPs should be appropriately expanded.

Grammar Tips

Task 1

1. June 27th, 1880; 2. me?; 3. example, Lily; 4. √; 5. life: a spacious; 6. √; 7. "Yes, I do."; 8. √; 9. kind-hearted; 10. √

Task 2

1. A; 2. D; 3. B; 4. C; 5. C; 6. B; 7. D; 8. A; 9. D; 10. A

Supplementary Reading

1. T; 2. F; 3. T; 4. T; 5. F

Vocabulary Tips

1. Immunotherapy; 2. self-destruct; 3. Immunoglobulin; 4. construct; 5. instruction

Unit 10

Translation for Reference

课文 A

"大健康"和中国医学的未来

所谓的第四次工业革命正在如火如荼地进行着，它带来了颠覆和机遇。具体来说，在医疗保健领域，数字化转型正在产生广泛而深刻的影响，带来了改变商业模式、服务、法规和技能供求的改变。

中国医疗领域的真空

中国政府的总体理念是从"以疾病为中心"的医疗转向"大健康"，旨在提供覆盖整个医疗连续体的全套医疗服务，重点是健康管理和慢性病管理。中国民众和卫生保健专业人员都认识到预防在卫生保健中的重要性。

不堪重负的基础设施

不堪重负的基础设施所承受的压力促使中国政府接受技术在减轻过度紧张的医疗体系负担方面的作用。其核心是鼓励大数据的应用，以实现精确诊断和个性化医疗。到2020年，将建立三个数字国家数据库，包括健康信息、健康档案和医疗记录。

智能设备和可穿戴设备的应用范围很广，可能会减少再入院的次数，提高急救反应的速度、提供更及时的护理以避免病情恶化或不良事件的发生，如中风、跌倒。

建立基于云的区域成像中心，支持低级医院确保首次正确诊断，连接不同级别的医院实现数据共享、远程咨询和双向转诊，这些只是数字技术将发挥关键作用的方式之一。

接受互联医疗

绝大多数（92%）的中国医疗专业人士认为，中国医疗体系的整合非常重要。幸运的是，政府几乎没有做什么来说服公众相信健康相关技术的好处：他们已经接受健康相关的应用，而且在很多情况下，已经在使用互联医疗技术来追踪他们自己的健康。

在从预防到诊断、从治疗到急性后护理的整个健康过程中，使用互联医疗技术的意愿将在创造更多更好的医疗解决方案方面发挥重要作用。

数字化转型

该领域的数字化转型潜力巨大——无论是在创造效率方面，还是在利用新机会改善患者结果方面。从联网的家庭和虚拟护理的进步，到数据驱动的解决方案，使患者的健康得到更有效的实时监测，数字解决方案有助于加速向基于价值的医疗保健的转变。

在预防和家庭护理方面尤其需要取得重大进展。从传统的以"医院内"开展治疗和健康护理为主，转变为在各种"院外环境"开展治疗和健康护理，不仅可以扩大治疗的地理区域和提高人群的人口多样性，而且也将标志着当前医疗模式的重大转变，释放出资源。

尽管，不可否认需要克服某些现有的结构性和文化障碍——从报销模式和财务激励到监管，甚至一些围绕信任的基本担忧——但中国政府已表现出接受这一转变的重大承诺。而且，正如一些活动已经证明的那样，智能、互联技术的广泛应用将继续提高人们看得起病的能力和增加看病的途径。

课文 B

药房自动化

药房自动化涉及日常药房工作的自动化。例如，配药、数据处理及处方的传统管理。

随着自动化和机器人技术的快速发展，研究人员正努力为药房管理提供广泛的解决方案。这些自动化解决方案范围从基本的药品分发和包装到更为复杂和高级的任务，如库存处理和财务管理。

药房自动化的优点

制药领域自动化和机器人技术的整合大大改善了药品分发的安全性、库存管理和标签功能。由人工智能和自动化带来的惊人的优点，甚至传统的装备也已经开始进行转变了。

（1）提高效率

自动化超越了最专注和专业的药剂师的专业技能和知识。特别是在精确度和速度方面，机器绝对是最安全的。除此之外，药房自动化还通过提高处方的总配药量，大大提高了生产效率，大大超过了药剂师过去靠手工工作所能达到的水平。

（2）减少药物浪费

使用最佳自动化操作的药剂师还可以控制灌装或贴标签过程中可能产生的潜在药物浪费。

（3）改善了咨询服务

药房自动化与减少药剂师的手工工作量密切相关。因此，药房工作人员可以更好地为病人提供咨询，回答他们的问题。

（4）降低劳动力成本

你知道吗？药剂师平均每天要在药房行走 8 英里左右的路程，做各种各样的药房工作。药房自动化使药剂师能够让正在进行的药房工作自动化，包括配处方药、贴标签和配药。药房自动化确保劳动力成本降低，也有助于减轻工作环境中的压力。

（5）保证安全

当药剂师配发受严格管制的药品时，药房区域发生人为错误就非常危险。例如，药房工作人员可以在语音邮件中提供机密信息，这可能危及公司或病人的安全或机密性。

药房可以通过整合自动化呼叫程序来显著降低这类风险，这些程序只为病人提供指令性信息。

药房自动化的趋势

（1）计数秤

计数秤是一种小型设备，可以安装在任何大小的药房。柜台带有条形码扫描仪，可以扫描标签和处方瓶。

（2）药片计数设备

药片计数工作配备了扫描仪和信息屏幕。这些设备可以让你检查标签和扫描药瓶，以确认配药正确。

除此之外，你还可以将药片计数工具与药房管理系统集成在一起，以简化工作流程并降低出错的风险。

（3）配药和包装机器人

配药和包装机器人根据要求执行不同的任务。部分配药机器人被用来读取处方，并从存储库中选择和分发正确的药物。类似地，部分机器人可以存储小瓶和标签。

另一方面，包装机器人被用来以一种智能的方式包装药片和药物，这样病人就不需要一个配药的工作人员来配取他们的常规药物了。

药房自动化已经改变了传统社区药房以往的工作方式。药房自动化使药房的工作流程合理化，提高了效率。

补充阅读

中国药膳

全世界许多人都喜欢吃中国菜。中国药膳是一种特殊类型的中国菜——一种值得你探索的古代治病艺术。它是一种传统中药。

药膳简介

正宗的药膳是根据传统的食谱和技术，基于人体运作的古老观念而制作的。他们描述各种肉类、谷物、草药或蔬菜对人体的影响，身体是如何运作的，并就如何保持健康或治疗疾病提出了建议。

最早的著作《黄帝内经》包含了中国食疗的基本思想，就不同的健康状况和不同的环境条件下应该吃什么提出了建议。

中国古代医学书籍列举了数百种植物、动物和化学成分，并介绍了它们对人体的具体作用。这些书籍介绍了人体健康有关的物理原理，并描述了草药或特殊食物如何帮助维持人体健康，以及艾灸和针灸等中医技术。

中国药膳的基本原理

（1）平衡

基本思想是平衡气和体液——中国传统医学的基础。人们认为，一个健康的身体或器官在气和体液方面具有适当的平衡。当它们失衡时，身体就会生病。

环境或身体伤害会破坏平衡。例如，寒冷的天气导致体内气虚或阴虚，所以应该吃高阳的食物。炎热的天气里，自然阳气过多，就应该吃高阴的食物。

（2）添加草药

有药效的草药或动物可以添加到饮食中治病。很多草药也被西医草药师和世界上其他地方的草药师用来治疗相同的病。因此这也充分表明草药能起到真正的药用效果。

（3）运用热和味

所有的食物按气分类，从高阳排到高阴。按五味分类，分为酸、甜、苦、辣、咸。食物的气和味能以其自己的方式影响身体。

一般认为人们应该在每顿饭中加入所有的口味并平衡热。大多数中国人认为，如果一种食物吃得太多，会导致身体失衡。

（4）用餐时的中医原理

古代文献不仅描述了准备什么饭菜，还描述了如何吃饭。可能你会对已经成为文化数百年之久的中国饮食习惯感到惊讶。

尽量避免过度加工的食物，吃原味食物。

吃时令蔬果。

一定确保将蔬菜煮熟再食用。

找个安静的地方坐下来吃饭。

充分地咀嚼食物。

慢慢地吃。

认真进食，远离干扰。在中医里，大脑对消化食物的好坏发挥着一定作用，所以要关注食物的味道。

不要遗漏每一餐。

午饭后，小憩一会儿。

References

[1] Ask the Scientists. The Basics of Traditional Chinese Medicine[EB/ OL]. [2020 – 08 – 09]. https://askthe scientists. com/traditional – chinese – medicine/

[2] Caring Ambassadors. Western Medicine[EB/OL]. [2020 – 08 – 11]. https://caringambassadors. org/healing /healthcare – options/western – medicine/

[3] Britannica kids. Human Disease [EB/OL]. [2020 – 08 – 18]. https://kids. britannica. com/students/article/human – disease/274019

[4] George A. Bender "*Great Moments in Pharmacy*". [M]. Detroit: Parke, Davis & Company ,1965:1 – 9.

[5] CollegeGrad. Pharmacists [EB/OL]. [2020 – 08 – 11]. https://collegegrad. com/careers/pharmacists.

[6] Ken Krizner. Hospital Pharmacist Role Expands in Patient Care[EB/ OL]. (2019 – 05 – 23) [2016 – 07 – 06]. https://www. managedhealthcareexecutive. com/view/hospital – pharmacist – role – expands – patient – care

[7] Michael Bihari, MD. Drug Classes [EB/OL]. (2020 – 03 – 26) [2020 – 03 – 26]. https://www. verywellhealth. com/drug – classes – 1123991.

[8] Pharmapproach. Prescription Drugs and Over – The – Counter Drugs: Do You Know the Difference? [EB/OL]. (20 20 – 03 – 30) [2020 – 03 – 26]. https://www. pharmapproach. com/prescription – drugs – and – over – the – counter – drugs/.

[9] apluscorp. Prescription Drugs Vs. OTCs: What's the Difference? [EB/OL]. (2017 – 03 – 22) [2017 – 03 – 22]. https:// www. aplususapharma. com/blog/prescription – vs – over – the – counter – drugs/.

[10] Alex. Chinese Medicine [EB/OL]. (2019 – 01 – 04) [2019 – 01 – 04]. https://www. xiahuang. vip /2019/01/04/ liuxue shenginchina_13/index. html.

[11] Miyo. I need to refill this prescription[EB/OL]. (2012 – 11 – 16) [2012 – 11 – 16]. http://talk. kekenet. com/show_ 499.

[12] Tingroom. Pharmacy – Health – Prescription [EB/OL]. (2018 – 04 – 02)[2018 – 04 – 02]. http://www. tingroom. com/ lesson/ept/427490. html.

[13] Byjus. Classification of Drugs [EB/OL]. https://byjus. com/chemistry/classification – drugs/.

[14] Gerenjianli. Personal Resume [EB/OL]. (2018 – 12 – 17) [2018 – 12 – 17]. http://www. gerenjianli. com/english/ ncvpnvcmq mmx . htm.

[15] Cao C and Brown B. (2019) Understanding Chinese medicine and western medicine to reach the maximum treatment benefit. J Transl Sci 6: DOI: 10. 15761/JTS. 1000334. [EB/OL]. (2019 – 05 – 03) [2019 – 05 – 03]. https://www. oatext. com/understanding – chinese – medicine – and – western – medicine – to – reach – the – maximum – treatment – benefit. php.

[16] Wikipedia. The Drug Development Process [EB/OL]. (2018 – 04 – 01) [2018 – 04 – 10]. http://www. fda. gov /patients/learn – about – drug – and – device – approvals/drug – development – process.

[17] Zongru Guo. Artemisinin anti – malarial drugs in China [EB/OL]. (2016 – 02 – 18)[2016 – 02 – 20]. https://www. ncbi. nlm. nih. gov/pmc/articles/PMC4788711/.

［18］Kara Rogers. Tu Youyou ［EB/OL］. （2019 - 10 - 07）［2019 - 10 - 10］. https：// www. britannica. com /biography/ Tu - Youyou.

［19］Jason Fernando. New Drug Application （NDA）［EB/OL］. （2020 - 05 - 01）. https：// www. investopedia. com/terms /n/new - drug - application - nda. asp.

［20］Olga Carroll. China's CFDA Drug and Biologics Regulatory Approval Process. New Trends and Pathways ［EB/OL］. （2017 - 03 - 24）. https：//www. linkedin. com/pulse/chinas - cfda - drug - biologics - regulatory - approval - new - carroll - ph - d -.

［21］James Chen. Investigational New Drug （IND）［EB/OL］. （2018 - 05 - 01）. https：// www. investopedia. com/ terms/i/investigational - new - drug - ind. asp.

［22］Abpi. Drug safety （pharmacovigilance）［EB/OL］. （2020）.［2020 - 09 - 10］. https：// www. abpi. org. uk/medicine - discovery/ building - a - thriving - environment - for - medicine - discovery/how - do - we - monitor - and - regulate medicines /drug - safety - pharmacovigilance/.

［23］Shan Juan. Overuse makes antibiotics anti - health.［EB/ OL］. China Daily. （2016 - 08 - 20）. ［2020 - 09 - 10］. https：//www. chinadaily. com. cn/opinion/2016 - 08/20/ content_26542769. htm.

［24］MedlinePlus. Drug Safety.［EB/ OL］. （2019 - 07 - 04）.［2020 - 09 - 10］. https：//medline-plus. gov/drugsafety. html

［25］Dailymed. Label：Tylenol Extra Strength - acetaminophen tablet, film coated.［EB/ OL］. （2020 - 07 - 16）.［2020 - 09 - 10］. https：//dailymed. nlm. nih. gov/dailymed/drugInfo. cfm? setid = 59773893 - 09a8 - 47a2 - 943a - e9ea9da4458a.

［26］Rita Milios. Everything You Need to Know About Over - the - Counter Drug Abuse.［EB/ OL］. National Rehabs Directory. （2019 - 11 - 04）.［2020 - 09 - 10］. https：//www. rehabs. com/pro - talk/everything - you - need - to - know - about - over - the - counter - drug - abuse/.

［27］Market to China. Chinese Online Pharmacy, A Bright Way To Sell Druugs［EB/OL］. （2018 - 05 - 04）［2020 - 08 - 04］. https：//www. marketingtochina. com/chinese - online - pharmacy - sell - drugs/.

［28］MBA Skool. Bayer Marketing Mix （4Ps） Strategy［EB/OL］. （2020 - 04 - 19）［2020 - 08 - 04］. https：// www. mbaskool. com/marketing - mix/products/16791 - bayer. html.

［29］Pharmacist. Pharmaceutical Industry Sales and Marketing［EB/OL］.［2020 - 08 - 04］https：// www. pharmacist. com/sites/default/files/files/Profile_25 _Pharmaceutical _Industry _Sales _Mar-keting_%20091813. pdf.

［30］Lembit Rago. Budiono Santoso. Drug Regulation：History, Present and Future.［M/CD］.［2008 -08］. https：// www. who. int/medicines/technical_briefing/tbs/Drug_Regulation _History_Present_Future. pdf .

［31］China NMPA/CFDA. China NMPA/CFDA - What You Must Know.［EB/ OL］.［2020 -08 -09］. https：// chinamed device. com/china - nmpa - cfda - questions - answers/china - nmpa - cfda - what - you - must - know/.

［32］China - Britain Business. China's Healthcare System.［EB/ OL］.［2020 - 08 - 27］. https：// focus. cbbc. org/how - china's - healthcare - system - actually - works/.

［33］U. S. Food& Drug Administration. An Introdcution to COVID - 19 Tests ［DB/OL］.［2020 - 08 -

29］. https://www. fda. gov/emergency – preparedness – and – response/coronavirus – disease – 2019 – covid – 19/covid – 19 – educational – resources.

［34］World Health Organization. Coronavirus disease（COVID – 19）［DB/OL］.（2020 – 06 – 15）［2020 – 08 – 29］. https://www. youtube. com/watch？v = i0ZabxXmH4Y.

［35］Andy Ho.‘Big health’and the future of medicine in China［EB/OL］.（2017 – 06 – 19）［2020 – 08 – 29］. https://www. weforum. org/agenda/2017/06/big – health – future – medicine – china/.

［36］Ronit Kappor. Pharmacy Automation，A Look at the Future of Pharmacy［EB/OL］.（2020 – 05 – 23）［2020 – 08 – 29］. https://thedigitalwise. com/2020/05/23/pharmacy – automation – a – look – at – the – future – of – pharmacy/.

［37］Gavin Van Hinsbergh. Chinese Medicinal Cuisine/ Food Therapy – Healthy Seasonal Recipes［EB/OL］.（2020 – 04 – 17）［2020 – 08 – 29］. https://www. chinahighlights. com/travelguide/chinese – food/medicinal – cuisine. htm.

［38］崔成红,李正亚. 医药英语［M］. 2 版. 北京:中国医药科技出版社,2017.

［39］史志祥. 药学英语(上册)［M］. 5 版. 北京:人民卫生出版社,2016.

［40］李有贵. 医药英语［M］. 北京:高等教育出版社,2012.

［41］孙路路. 国家执业药师职业资格考试指南·药学专业知识(二)［M］. 8 版. 北京:中国医药科技出版社,2020.

［42］陈美华,郭锋萍. 医药英语教程［M］. 北京:高等教育出版社,2011.

［43］常光萍. 医药英语［M］. 2 版. 北京:中国医药科技出版社,2016.

［44］刘彦,潘伦,何坪,等. 2015 ~ 2018 年重庆市毕业后全科医生教育开展情况研究［J］. 中国全科医学,2020,23(19):2374 – 2378.

［44］成撒诺,何坪,邓宇等. 重庆市基本公共卫生服务绩效考核指标体系构建研究［J］. 中国全科医学,2018,21(10):1161 – 1166.